Minimally Invasive (Endoscopic & Robotic) Breast Surgery

Minimally Invasive (Endoscopic & Robotic) Breast Surgery

Hung-Wen Lai, MD, PhD

Director of the Endoscopic and Oncoplastic Breast Surgery Center
Division of General Surgery
Department of Surgery
Changhua Christian Hospital
Changhua, Taiwan

Chi Wei Mok, MBBS, MMED, FRCSEd

Consultant Oncoplastic and Minimally Invasive (MIS)
Endoscopic & Robotic Breast Surgeon
Division of Breast Surgery
Department of Surgery
Changi General Hospital
Singapore
Consultant
Singhealth Duke-NUS Breast Centre
Singapore

ELSEVIER

Elsevier
Radarweg 29, PO Box 211, 1000 AE Amsterdam, Netherlands
The Boulevard, Langford Lane, Kidlington, Oxford OX5 1GB, United Kingdom
50 Hampshire Street, 5th Floor, Cambridge, MA 02139, United States

Notices

Practitioners and researchers must always rely on their own experience and knowledge in evaluating and using any information, methods, compounds or experiments described herein. Because of rapid advances in the medical sciences, in particular, independent verification of diagnoses and drug dosages should be made. To the fullest extent of the law, no responsibility is assumed by Elsevier, authors, editors or contributors for any injury and/or damage to persons or property as a matter of products liability, negligence or otherwise, or from any use or operation of any methods, products, instructions, or ideas contained in the material herein.

ISBN: 978-0-323-73405-9

Publisher: Cathleen Sether
Acquisition Editor: Belinda Kuhn
Editorial Project Manager: Susan Ikeda
Production Project Manager: Poulouse Joseph
Cover Designer: Alan Studholme

To my wife, Ling-Tzu Huang, *who has always accepted me for who I am and supported my hustle, drive, and ambition: you are and always will be my perfect wife and mother to our children.*

To my children, Yuan-Chieh Lai, Po-Yuan Lai, and Pin-Hsin Lai and my great-great-great-grandchildren who I will never have the pleasure of meeting: I want you to know where you came from.

Dr. Hung-Wen Lai, MD, PHD

For my ever-supportive wife, Fang Yu and lovely son, baby KJ.
For my mentor in surgery, Professor Su-Ming Tan.
And most importantly, my patients who have shown remarkable determination and taught me the meaning of life!

Dr. Chi Wei Mok, MBBS, FRCSEd

Contents

SECTION 3 Endoscopic mastectomy with immediate reconstruction

PART 2 Robotic breast surgery

SECTION 1 Robotic breast surgery with no reconstruction

SECTION 2 Robotic breast surgery with reconstruction

Acknowledgements

I would like to express my special thanks of gratitude to my **Mentors: Shou-Jen Kuo, Shou-Tung Chen, Dar-Ren Chen, Jean Yves Petit and Eisuke Fukuma** who taught me a lot and gave me the golden opportunity to do this wonderful project **'Minimal Invasive (Endoscopic & Robotic) Breast Surgery'**, which also helped me in doing a lot of Research and I came to know about so many new things I am really thankful to them.

Second, I would also like to thank my parents (Hsi-Ching Lai and Hui-Yen Lai Hsu), friends and assistants who helped me a lot in finalizing this project within the limited time frame.

Dr. Hung-Wen Lai, MD, PHD

I have to start by thanking my awesome wife, Fang Yu. From reading my early drafts to giving suggestions on the contents and most importantly keeping our little munchkin KJ occupied so I could concentrate on writing, she is equally important in getting this book published as I was. Thank you so much, my dear!

I would also like to thank my parents Phillip and Ivy, siblings Jason, Stanley and Mazel for giving me an awesome family as well as my in laws Kent and Joyce for nurturing a lovely daughter in Fang Yu.

Equally important in nurturing me to who I am today, my mentor in surgery Professor Su-Ming Tan and my mentor in minimally invasive breast surgery Dr. Hung-Wen Lai.

A million thanks to my fellow consultants, breast care nurses and support staffs from Breast Centre@Changi & Division of Breast Surgery, Department of Surgery, Changi General Hospital, Singapore for their awesome camaraderie and support.

Heartfelt thanks to the marvellous team from Dr. Hung-Wen Lai's research group (Yun-Ting Chang, Yi-Ru Ke, Shun-Ying Tsai, Shu-Hsin Pai, Chin-Mei Tai) for their great assistance in record-keeping, maintaining the cancer database and excellent photography.

Last but not the least, Belinda, Susan and everyone else at the Elsevier team for making this book a reality!

Dr. Chi Wei Mok, MBBS, FRCSEd

Introduction

Breast conservation surgery has taken a change in paradigm in recent years. From conventional breast conservation surgery to oncoplastic breast surgery, the breast surgery community has witnessed the advent of surgical techniques aiming at improving cosmetic outcomes while maintaining oncological safety in the surgical management of breast cancer.

Minimally invasive breast surgery, a term coined and popularized over a decade ago, has been the leading forefront of surgical innovations in the field of breast cancer surgery. Endoscopic or video-assisted and robotic breast surgery in particular has been gaining popularity over the past few years owing to the attractive concept of performing oncological resection with small or inconspicuously placed surgical incisions.

In this book *Minimally Invasive (Endoscopic & Robotic) Breast Surgery: A Guide to Clinical Practice*, various minimally invasive breast surgery techniques along with reconstruction options after breast conserving surgery or mastectomy were presented in a sequential manner from preoperative markings to intraoperative and postoperative pictures with discussion by the authors on the technical know-how, tips as well as potential complications.

This book comes at a right time to serve as a guide to breast and plastic surgeons interested in performing minimally invasive breast surgery, as there have been little resources offering pictorial guides of extensive lists of minimally invasive techniques through case discussions. The authors hope that a myriad of minimally invasive techniques showcased through an easy to follow format with case discussions will encourage more surgeons to adopt these techniques and improve the cosmetic outcomes of patients with breast cancer.

Hung-Wen Lai, MD, PhD
Division of General Surgery
Department of Surgery
Changhua Christian Hospital
135, Nanhsiao Street, Changhua 500, Taiwan
Phone no: +886-4-723-8595 ext.4881, FAX: +886-4-723-3715
E-mail: hwlai650420@yahoo.com.tw; 143809@cch.org.tw

Chi Wei Mok, MBBS, FRCSEd
Division of Breast Surgery
Department of Surgery
Changi General Hospital
2 Simei Street 3 Singapore 529889
Email address: mok.chi.wei@singhealth.com.sg

PART

1

Endoscopic or video-assisted breast surgery

SECTION

1

Endoscopic breast surgery with no reconstruction

CHAPTER 1

Endoscopic breast-conserving surgery

Description of technique

Pre-operative marking and positioning

Pre-operative marking was done with the patient in standing and supine position. After induction of general anaesthesia, the patient was then placed in supine position and ipsilateral arm abducted to 90 degrees to avoid affecting the operative procedure. Endoscopic video monitors (Olympus Optical Co., Tokyo, Japan) were set up on both sides of the patient's head to allow both the surgeon and assistant to view the monitor. An oblique-ended rigid endoscope measuring 5 mm in diameter with a viewing angle of 30 degrees was used in all procedures.

Axillary staging procedure

In patients for whom sentinel lymph node biopsy (SLNB) is indicated, a small amount (2−3 mCi) of radioisotope Tc99m was injected intradermally at the site of the tumour before operation (either on the day or 1 day prior).

After induction of general anaesthesia, 3 mL of 1% methylene blue (Merck, Darmstadt, Germany) was injected into the breast parenchyma in equally divided aliquots at five positions surrounding the hemisphere of the tumour facing the ipsilateral axilla. The breast tissue from the tumour to the axilla was then gently massaged for 5−10 minutes. Within 20−30 minutes after injection of the blue dye, a handheld gamma probe (Navigator; USSC, Norwalk, CT) was used to identify hot spots and the location of the hottest nodes was then marked. An approximately 3-cm oblique axillary incision was then made close to the hottest nodes, and SLNB was then performed. Fresh frozen section was performed as indicated. If SLNB was positive for metastases, a complete axillary lymph node dissection up to level II was performed.

Dissection of breast parenchyma off pectoralis major fascia

After completion of axillary staging procedure, dissection was carried out to the lateral border of the pectoralis major muscle. The margin between pectoralis muscle and breast parenchyma was clearly identified. An endoscopic Ultra Retractor (Johnson & Johnson KK or Karl Storz) vein harvester was used for the dissection pectoral

Minimally Invasive (Endoscopic & Robotic) Breast Surgery. https://doi.org/10.1016/B978-0-323-73405-9.00001-7

muscle fascia off posterior portion of breast parenchyma. The penetrating vessels were coagulated and cut with bipolar scissors (PowerStar, Johnson & Johnson KK) or a harmonic scalpel to ensure adequate haemostasis and therefore better visual clarity. Counter traction was applied by retracting surrounding tissue with the Ultra Retractor under endoscopic guidance to create a sufficient working space, and a suction tube can be used to evacuate mist and smoke.

Tunnelling and development of skin flap

After completion of the axillary staging procedure, a semi-circular peri-areolar skin incision or a single axillary incision was made (depending on surgeon's preference) as previously described. A physiological saline solution containing lidocaine 0.05% and epinephrine 1:1,000,000 was injected subcutaneously into the whole breast to minimize bleeding. An approximately 3–5-mm-thick skin flap was created via tunnelling method using an optical bladeless trocar Xcel (Johnson & Johnson, Tokyo, Japan) under endoscopic guidance. Subsequently, the septa between the skin flap and parenchyma was dissected and taken off under endoscopic guidance using endoscissors, bipolar scissors, or a harmonic scalpel.

Performing wide excision and repair of resection cavity

After development of adequate skin flap (either via a single axillary or combination of axillary and peri-areolar incision, wide excision was performed using bipolar or monopolar diathermy). To guide resection with adequate margins, the authors recommended the use of intra-operative ultrasound and marking of resection margin with blue dye injection. Specimen was retrieved thereafter and haemostasis secured. Level I oncoplastic techniques were used to approximate breast parenchyma and drain was placed on a case-to-case basis.

Case 1: endoscopic breast-conserving surgery

Patient/demographics

This is a case of a 40-year-old lady with a 1.3-cm tumor in the left upper outer quadrant. Core biopsy pre-operatively revealed an invasive ductal carcinoma, ER/PR positive, CerbB2 positive. Metastatic workup was negative. The patient opted for breast conservation, and she was not keen for any form of reconstruction.

Surgery and pathology report

The patient underwent an endoscopic-assisted breast-conserving surgery with sentinel lymph node biopsy via a single axillary incision. The frozen section for the sentinel lymph node biopsy was negative, and final routine histopathology revealed a T1cN0 (0/4 LN)M0 tumor with clear margins.

Post-operative outcomes

There were no immediate post-operative complications, and the patient was discharged well. In addition, she was reviewed in the outpatient clinic with satisfactory reporting of her cosmetic outcomes. She subsequently had adjuvant radiotherapy as well as endocrine therapy for 5 years.

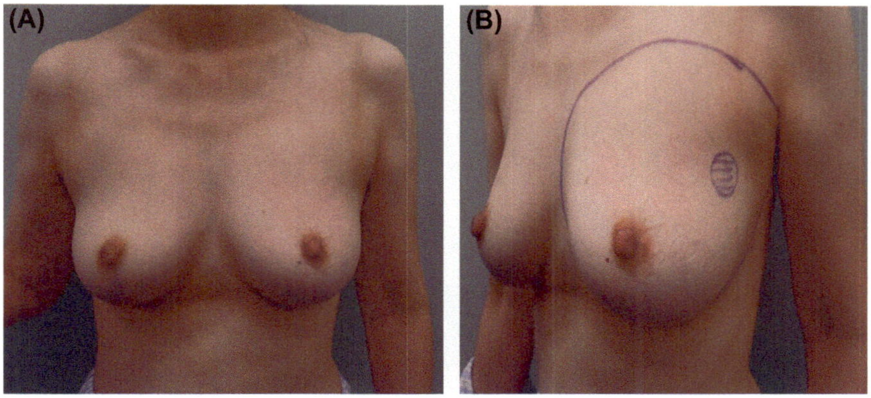

1.1A, 1B

Pre-operative front and lateral view showing location of tumor in the left upper outer quadrant.

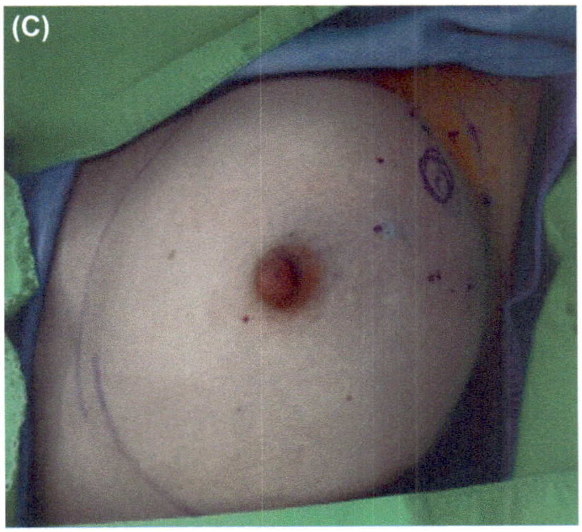

1.1C

Localization of tumor with methylene blue dye under intra-operative ultrasound guidance.

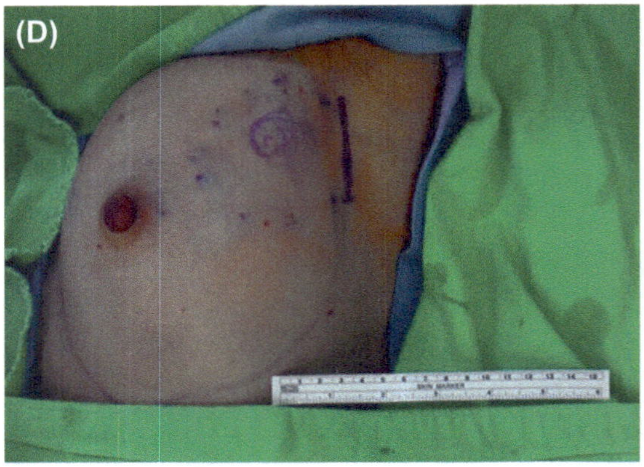

1.1D

Single axillary incision planned for the wide excision.

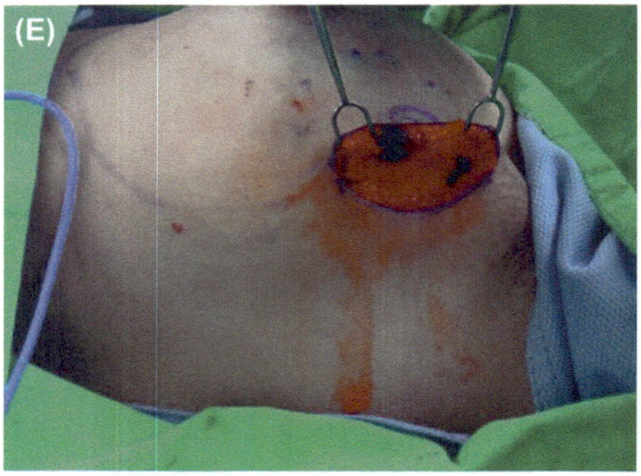

1.1E

Raising of skin flap after sentinel lymph node biopsy.

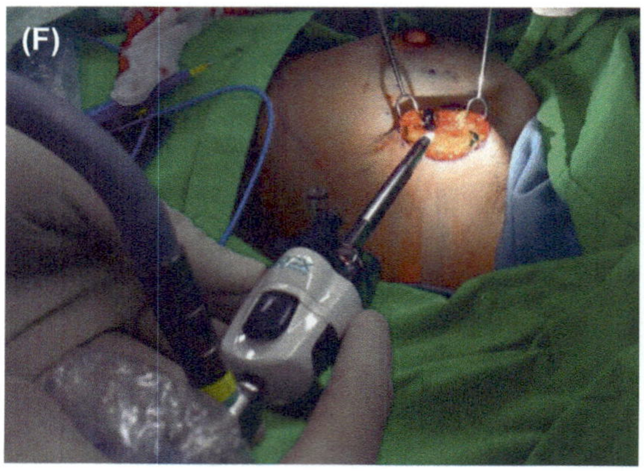

1.1F

Tunneling technique in raising skin flap demonstrated here with bladeless Optical trocar.

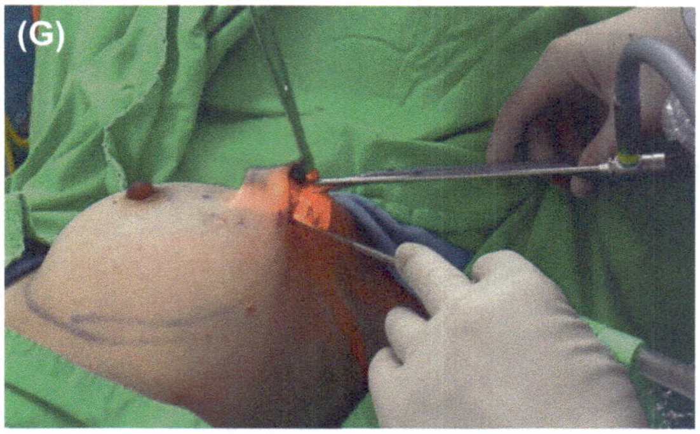

1.1G

Under endoscopic visualization, septa between skin flap and breast parenchyma was taken off with bipolar scissors.

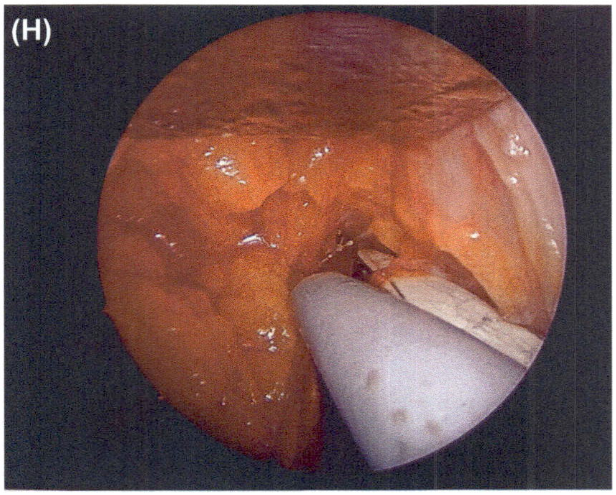

1.1H

Endoscopic view showing dissection of skin flap.

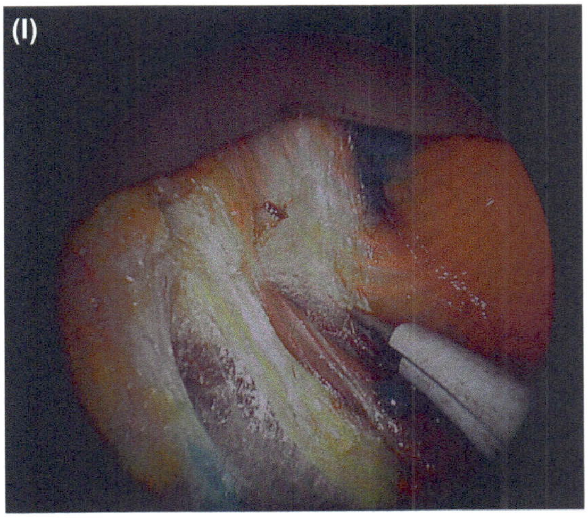

1.1I

Endoscopic view showing dissection of breast parenchyma off pectoralis major fascia.

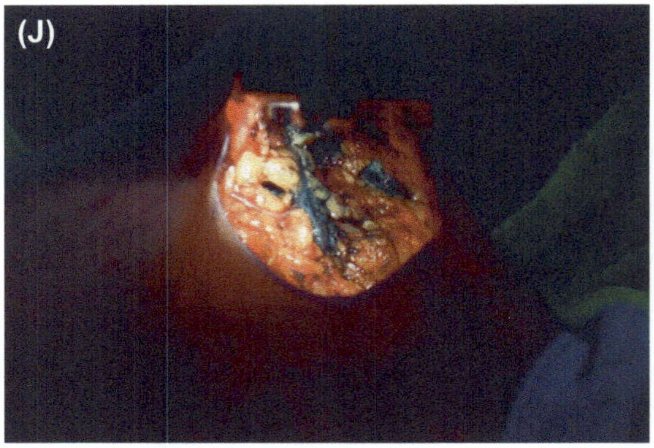

1.1J

Direct view of the resection cavity showing blue dye marking of margins over the breast parenchyma.

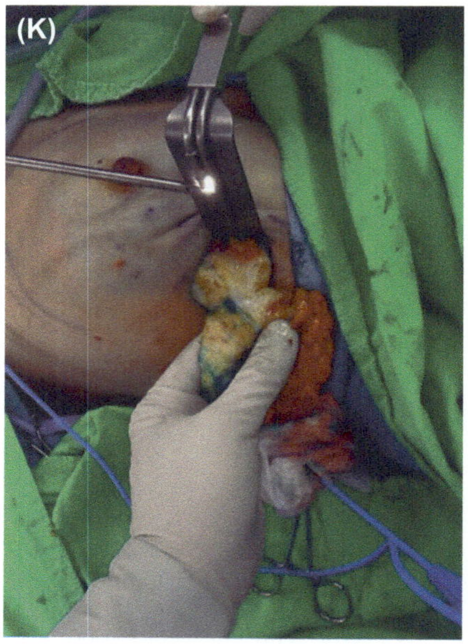

1.1K

Delivering specimen via axillary incision.

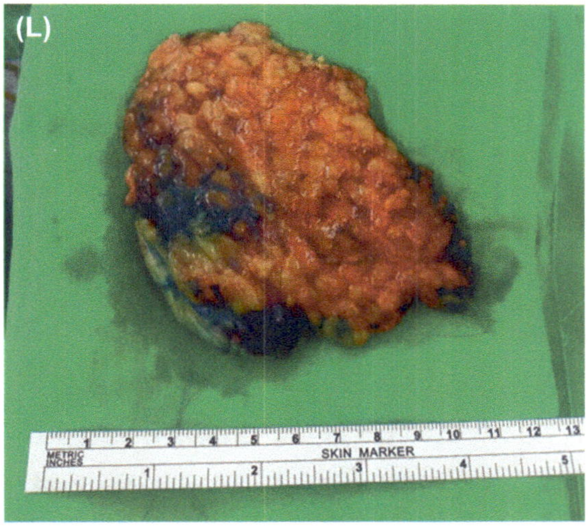

1.1L

Wide excision specimen removed intact.

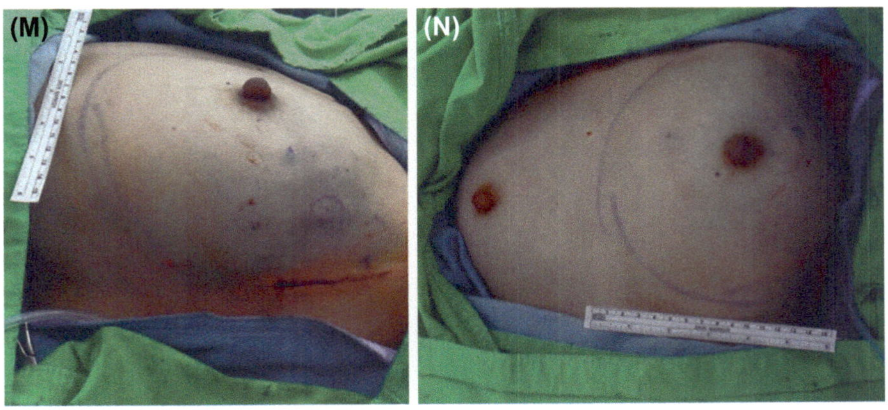

1.1M, N

Immediate post-operative lateral and front view showing axillary incision that was well hidden.

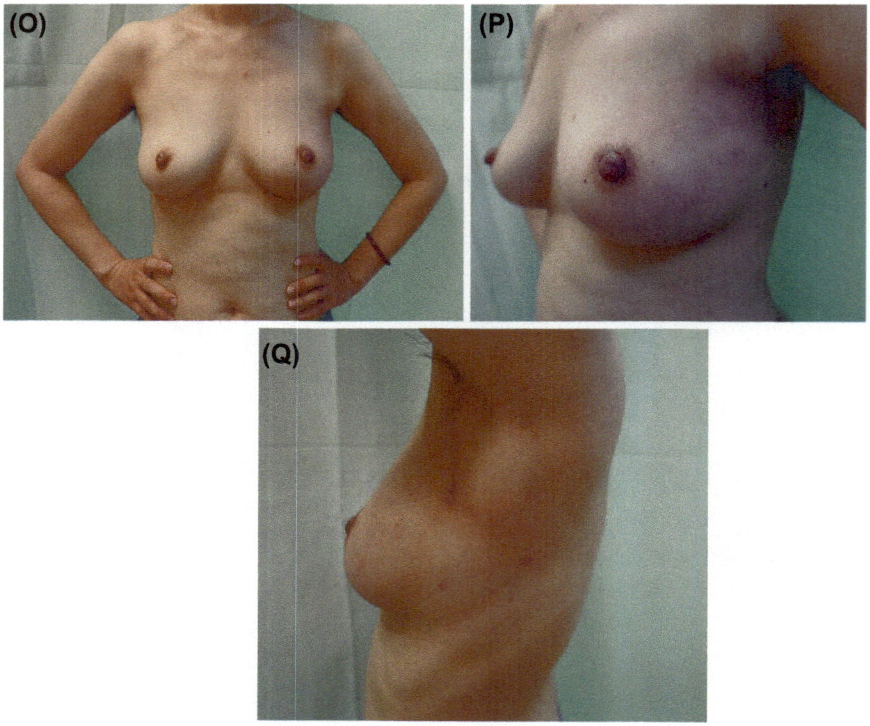

1.10–Q

Front and lateral views showing well-hidden and well-healed scar with excellent cosmesis (2 months post-operative).

Case 2: endoscopic breast-conserving surgery

Patient/demographics

The second case described a 51-year-old lady diagnosed with clinical stage I right breast cancer with a pre-operative core biopsy report of an invasive lobular carcinoma with lobular carcinoma in situ ER+, PR+, and CerbB2+. The tumor was located at the right upper inner quadrant, approximately 6.8 cm from the nipple as shown in her pre-operative magnetic resonance imaging (MRI).

Her metastatic workup did not reveal any distant metastases. The patient opted for a wide excision, and she was not keen for reconstruction.

Surgery and pathology report

The patient underwent an endoscopic-assisted breast-conserving surgery with sentinel lymph node biopsy. The operation was performed via an axillary and peri-areolar incision in view of the tumor location. Intra-operative frozen section of the sentinel lymph nodes revealed metastatic carcinoma and patient subsequently underwent axillary dissection up to level II axillary lymph nodes. Final histopathology revealed a multifocal T1cN1(1/17)M0, stage IIA disease with clear margins.

Post-operative outcomes

The patient was discharged well with no immediate complications encountered. She subsequently received adjuvant endocrine therapy for 5 years but declined adjuvant radiotherapy. The patient and surgeon verbalized satisfaction over post-op cosmesis.

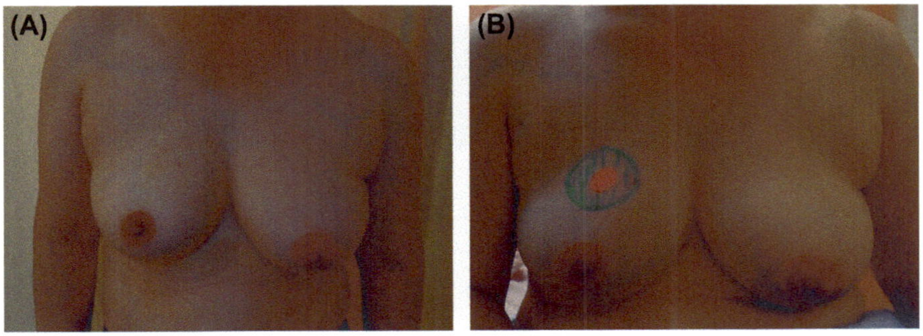

1.2A, B

Pre-operative front views showing location of tumor in the right upper inner quadrant.

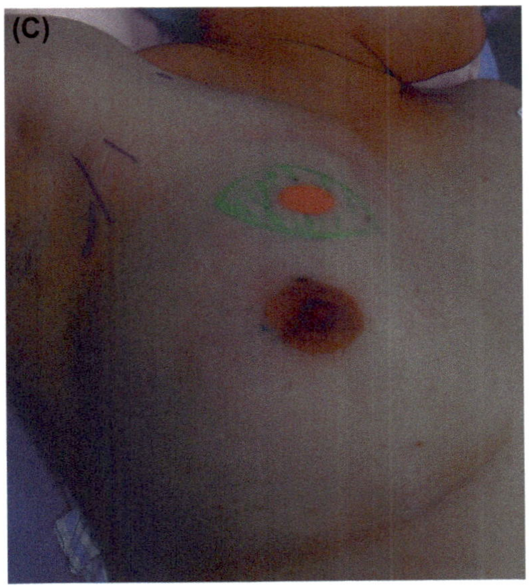

1.2C

On-table view of tumor in relation to the planned incisions (axilla and peri-areolar).

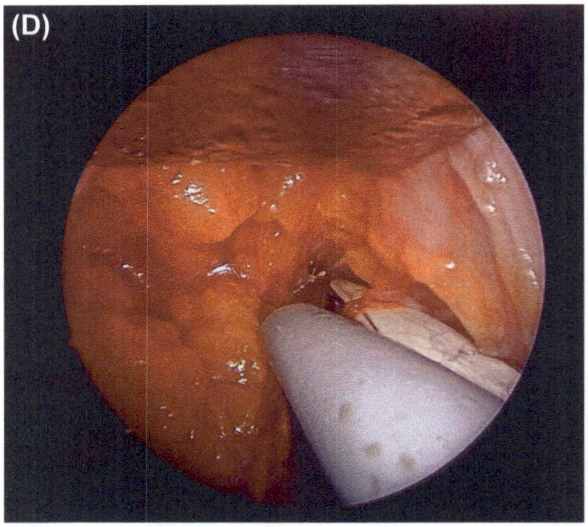

1.2D

Endoscopic view showing dissection of skin flap with bipolar scissors.

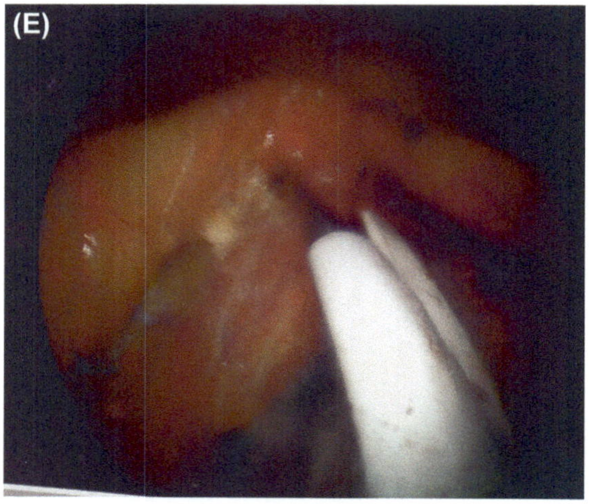

1.2E

Intra-operative endoscopic view showing dissection of breast parenchyma off pectoralis major fascia.

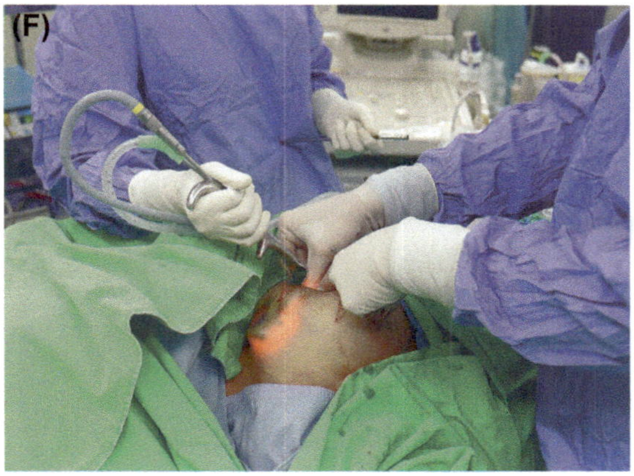

1.2F

Use of lighted retractor to aid in retraction and visualization during wide excision.

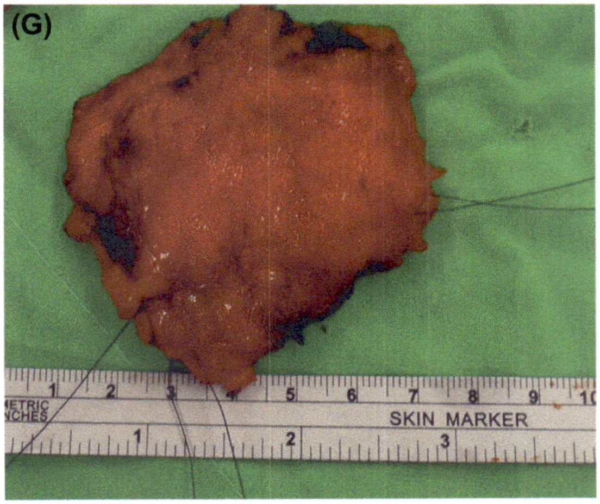

1.2G

Specimen removed intact and oriented appropriately.

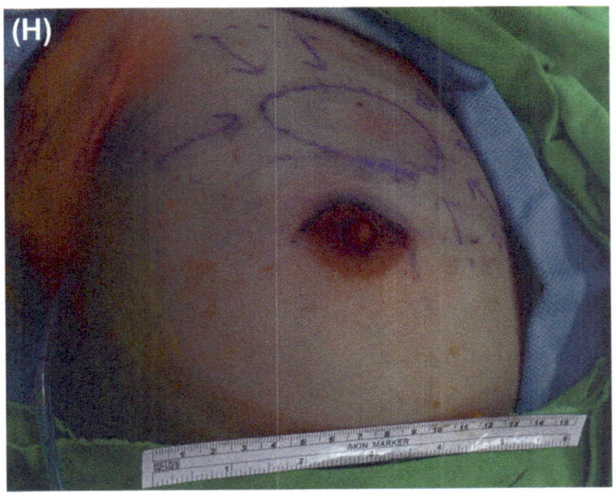

1.2H

Immediate post-operative view showing inconspicuous incisions in the axilla and peri-areolar region.

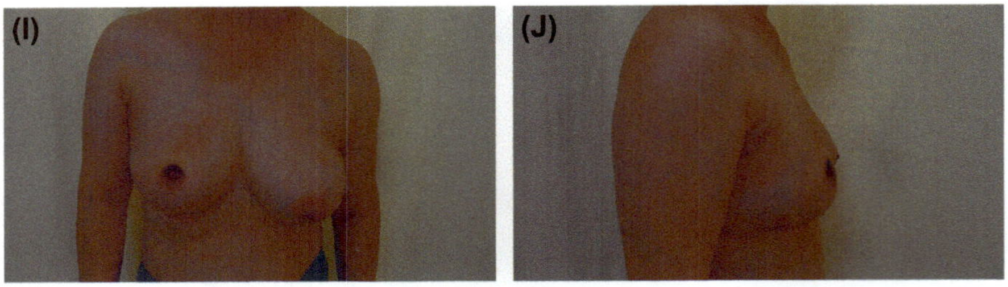

1.21, J

1 month post-operative front and lateral views showing a well-healed scar that was barely visible. Of note, patient had asymmetry of both breasts pre-operatively and no significant change was noted post-op.

Case 3: endoscopic breast-conserving surgery – single peri-areolar incision

Patient/demographics

This case described a 50-year-old lady diagnosed with clinical stage I left breast cancer with a pre-operative core biopsy report of an invasive ductal carcinoma with ductal carcinoma in situ ER+, PR+, and CerbB2 negative. The tumor was located in the left upper outer quadrant.

Her metastatic workup did not reveal any distant metastases. The patient opted for breast conservation with no reconstruction.

Surgery and pathology report

The patient underwent an endoscopic-assisted breast-conserving surgery with sentinel lymph node biopsy. The operation was performed via a single peri-areolar incision. Intra-operative frozen section of the sentinel lymph nodes revealed no evidence of metastatic carcinoma. Final histopathology revealed a T1bN0M0, stage IA disease with clear margins.

Post-operative outcomes

The patient was discharged well with no immediate complications encountered. She subsequently received adjuvant radiotherapy as well as 5 years of endocrine therapy.

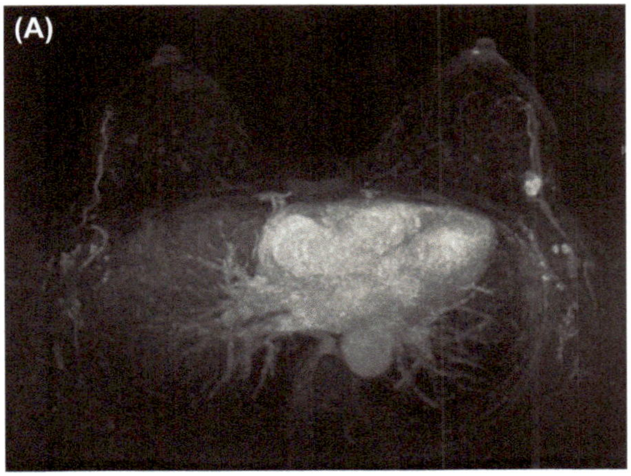

1.3A

Pre-operative MRI image showing location of tumor in the upper outer quadrant.

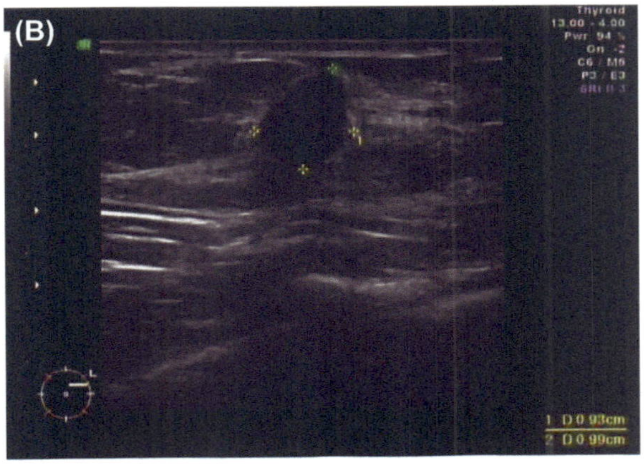

1.3B

Pre-operative ultrasound image showing a taller than wider, irregular nodule measuring 0.9 × 0.9 cm.

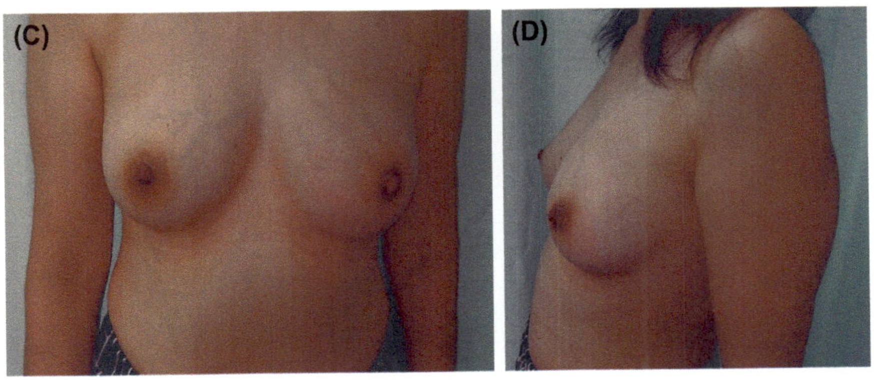

1.3C, D

Pre-operative front and lateral views of the patient.

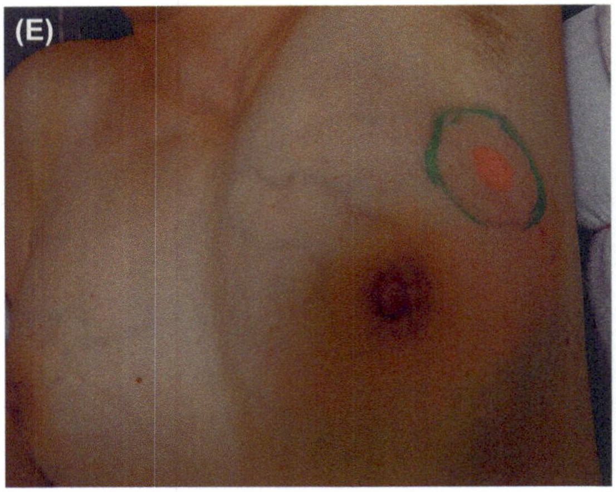

1.3E

On-table view showing the location of tumor with wire localization performed.

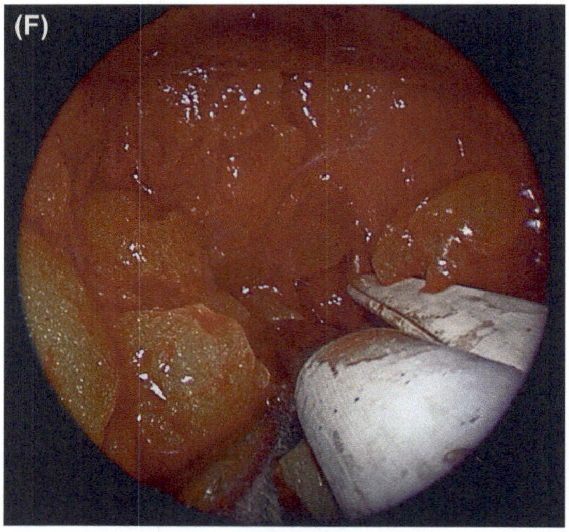

1.3F

Endoscopic view showing dissection of skin flap with bipolar scissors.

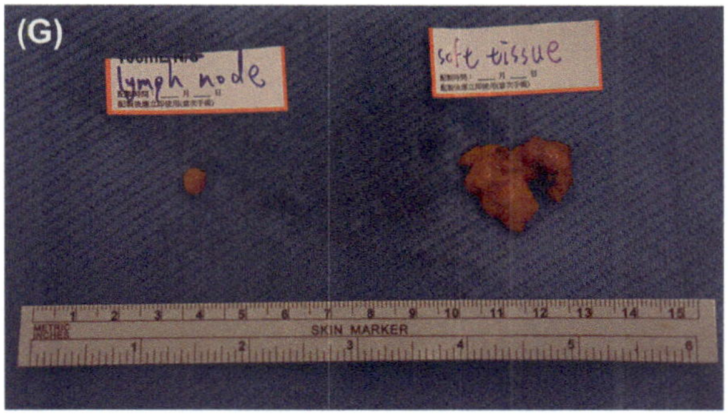

1.3G

Sentinel lymph node and axillary tissue sent for intra-operative frozen section analysis.

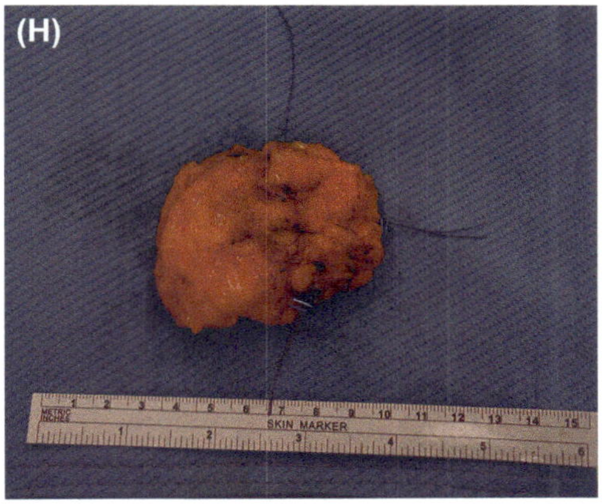

1.3H

Wide excision specimen removed intact and oriented with silk sutures.

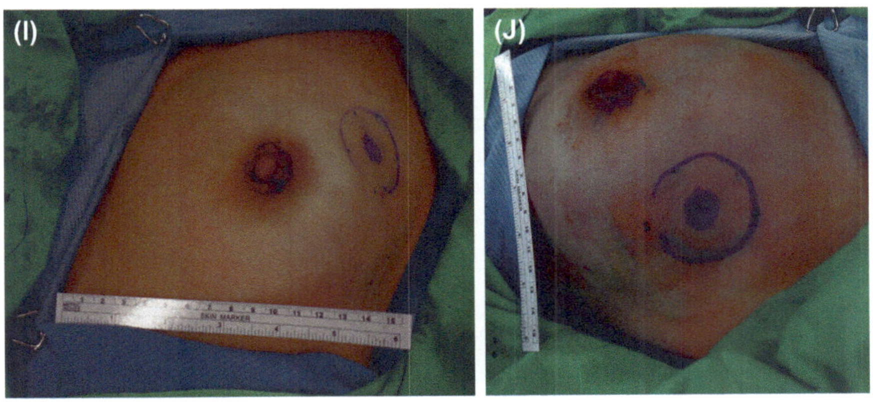

1.3I, J

Immediate post-operative views showing inconspicuous incisions in the peri-areolar region.

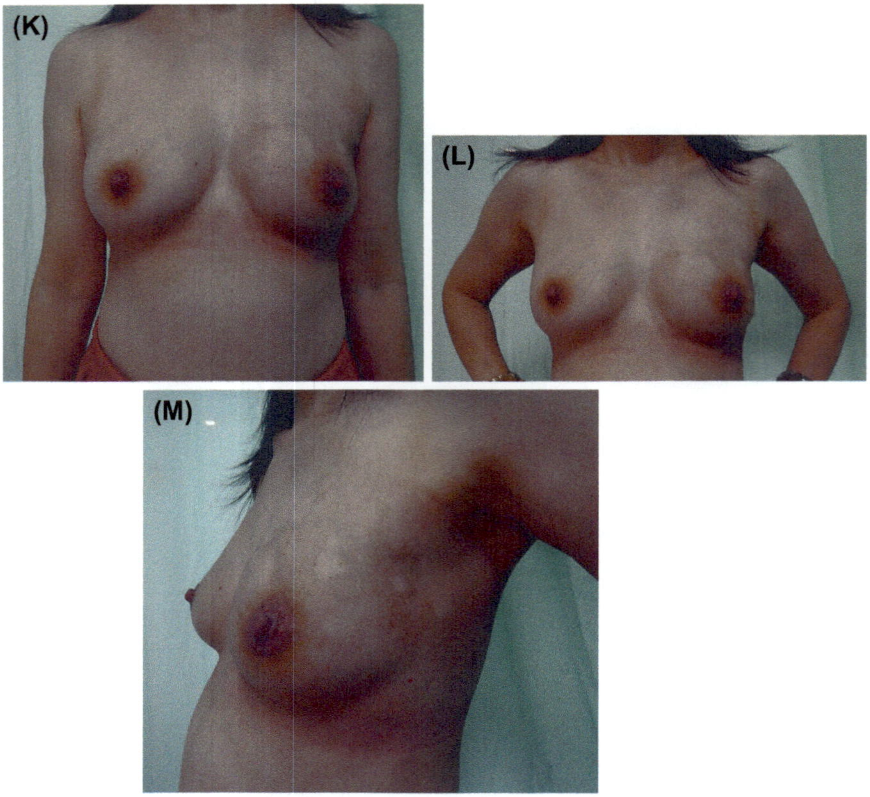

1.3K–3M

3 months post-operative front and lateral views showing a well-healed scar that was barely visible. Post-radiotherapy changes were also noted.

Case 4: endoscopic breast-conserving surgery – single areolar incision

Patient/demographics

This is a case of a 43-year-old lady with a 1-cm tumor in the right upper outer quadrant. Core biopsy pre-operatively revealed an invasive tubular carcinoma, ER, PR positive, and CerbB2 negative. Metastatic workup was negative. The patient was counseled and decided for endoscopic breast conserving surgery with no reconstruction.

Surgery and pathology report

The patient underwent an endoscopic-assisted wide excision with sentinel lymph node biopsy. The frozen section for the sentinel lymph node biopsy was negative, and final routine histopathology revealed a T1cN0(0/1LN)M0, stage 1A disease with uninvolved margins.

Post-operative outcomes

There were no immediate post-operative complications, and the patient was discharged well. She was subsequently reviewed in the outpatient clinic with satisfactory reporting of her aesthetic outcomes. She subsequently had adjuvant radiotherapy as well as endocrine therapy for 5 years.

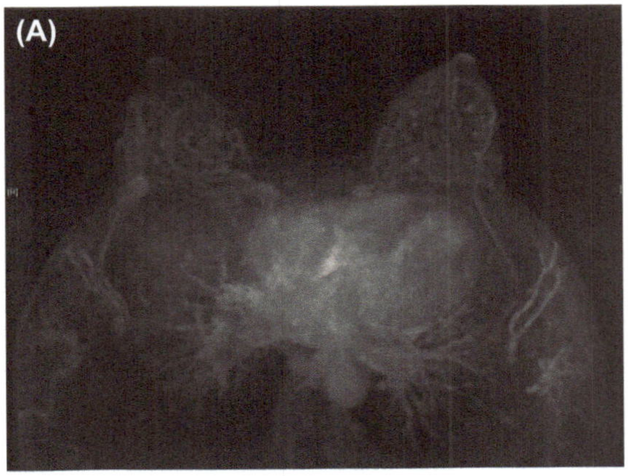

1.4A

Pre-operative MRI image showing location of tumor in the right upper outer quadrant.

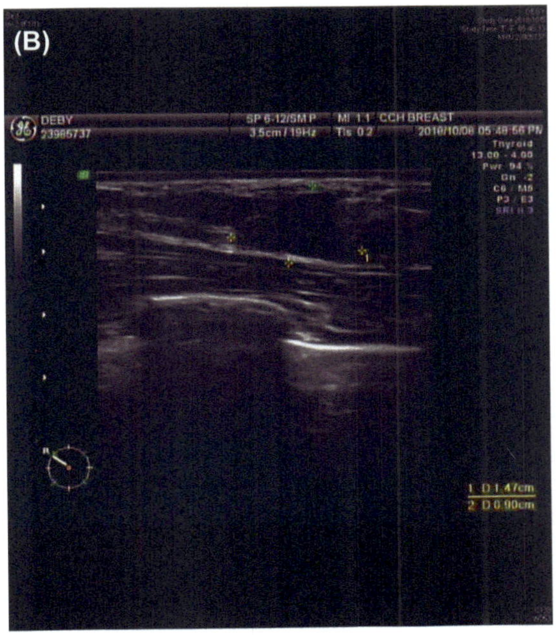

1.4B

Pre-operative ultrasound image showing location of tumor in the right upper outer quadrant with a size of 1.4 × 0.9 cm.

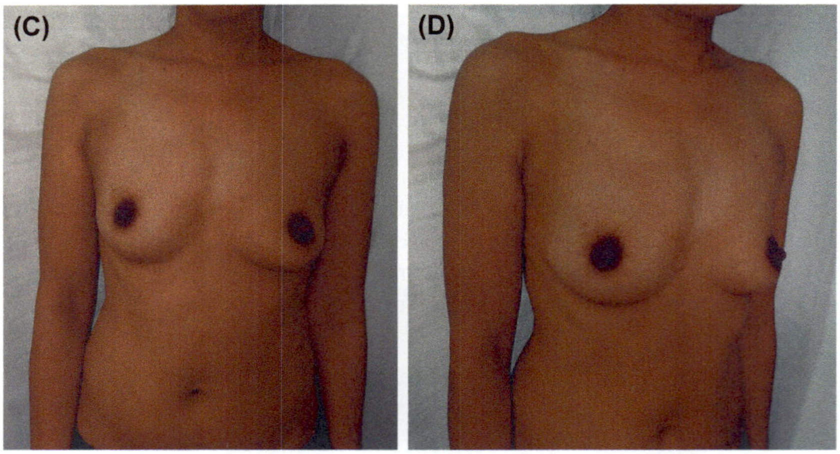

1.4C, 4D

Pre-operative front and lateral views of the patient. Of note, patient's left breast is relatively more ptotic if compared to the right side.

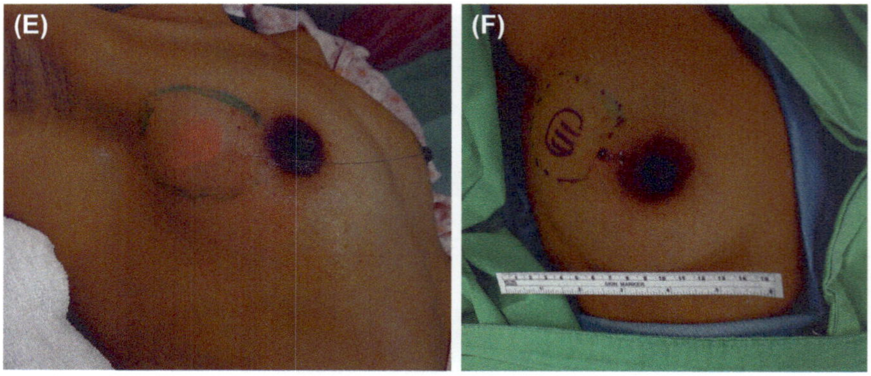

1.4E, F

On-table front and lateral views showing the location and wire localization of the tumor.

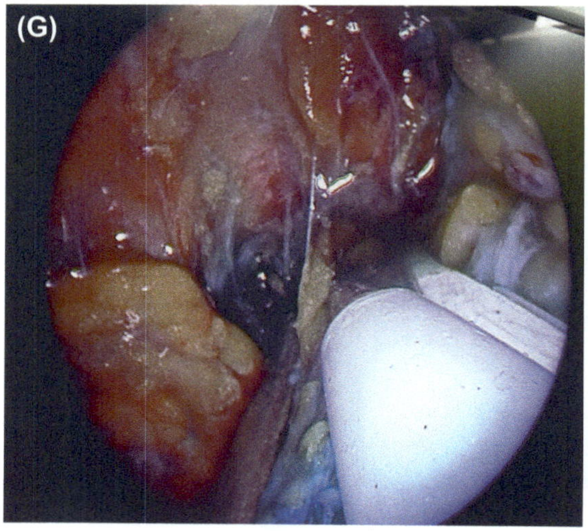

1.4G

Under endoscopic visualization, septa between skin flap and breast parenchyma was taken off with bipolar scissors.

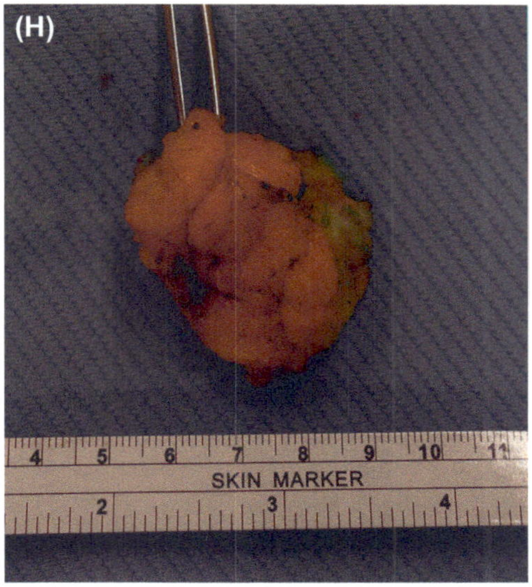

1.4H

Wide excision specimen removed intact – picture taken before orientation.

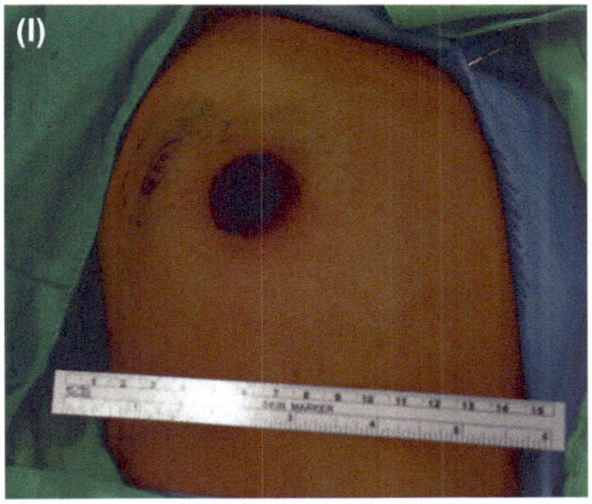

1.4I

Immediate post-operative front view showing a well-hidden peri-areolar incision.

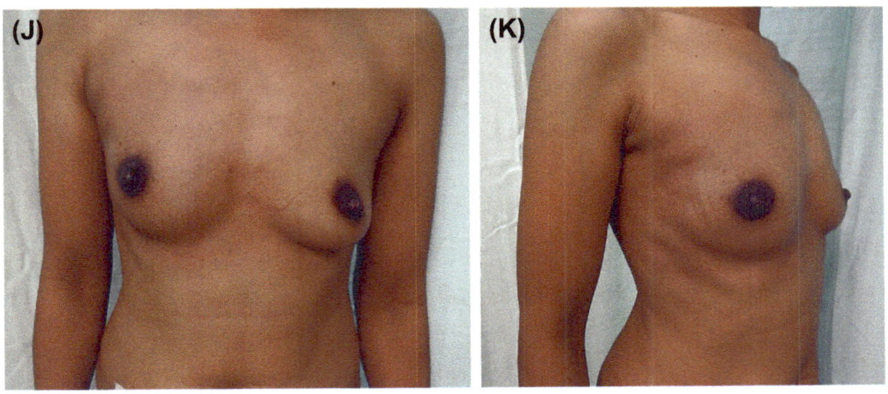

1.4J, K

Front and lateral views showing well-hidden and well-healed scar with excellent cosmesis (6 months post-operative views).

Case 5: endoscopic breast-conserving surgery – dual incision (inframammary fold and peri-areolar)

Patient/demographics

This case described a 61-year-old lady presented with a screen-detected right breast nodule measuring 1 cm and a pre-operative core biopsy report of a ductal carcinoma in situ. The tumor was located near the inframammary fold at six o'clock position.

The patient was counseled and agreeable for endoscopic breast-conserving surgery and sentinel lymph node biopsy.

Surgery and pathology report

The patient underwent an endoscopic-assisted breast-conserving surgery with sentinel lymph node biopsy. The operation was performed via dual incision (inframmary and axilla incision). Intra-operative frozen section of the sentinel lymph nodes revealed no evidence of metastatic carcinoma. Final histopathology revealed residual classical lobular carcinoma in situ with no invasive component.

Post-operative outcomes

The patient was discharged well with no immediate complications encountered. She reported excellent satisfaction in terms of aesthetic outcomes and did not receive any adjuvant therapy. Instead, she was on high-risk surveillance in view of her history of LCIS.

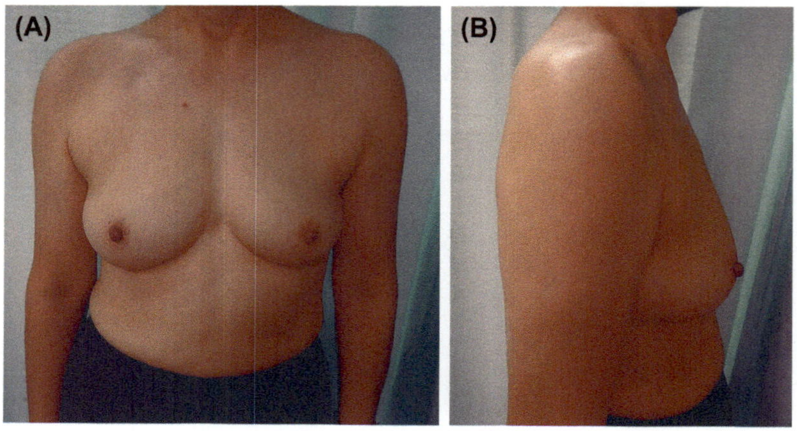

1.5A, B

Pre-operative front and lateral views of the patient.

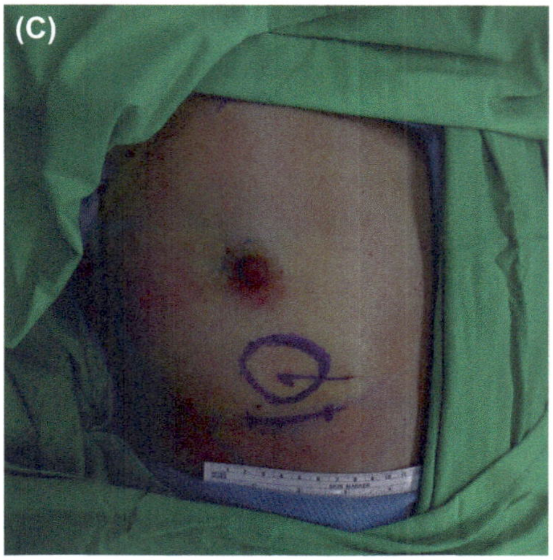

1.5C

On-table view showing the location of tumor with wire localization performed.

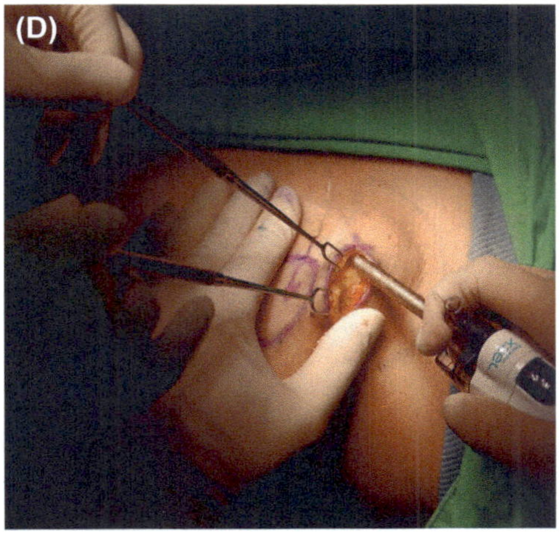

1.5D

Subcutaneous tunneling before skin flap dissection.

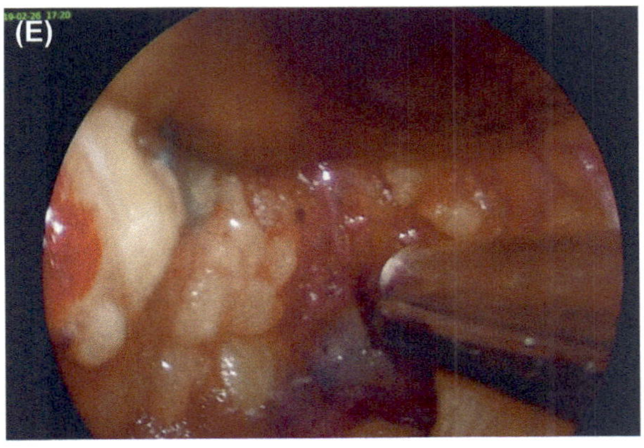

1.5E

Endoscopic view showing skin flap dissection with monopolar diathermy.

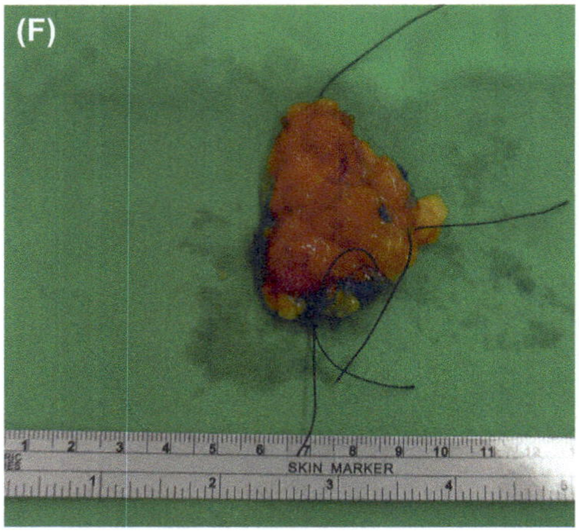

1.5F

Wide excision specimen removed intact and oriented with silk sutures.

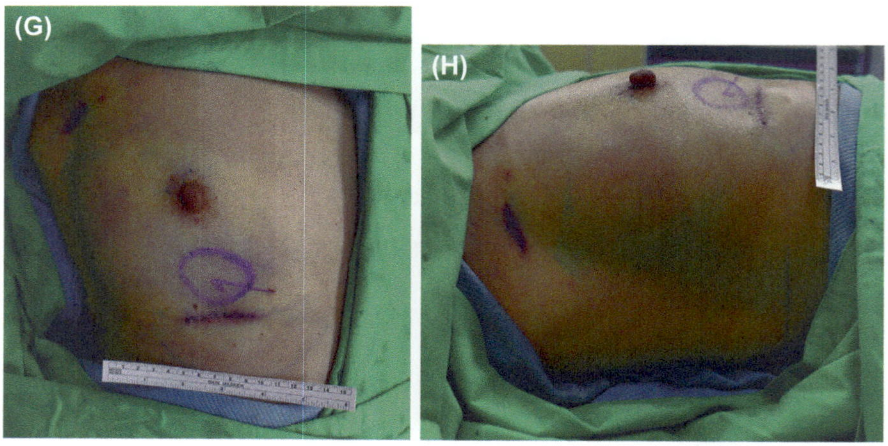

1.5G, H

Immediate post-operative views showing inconspicuous incisions in the inframammary and peri-areolar regions.

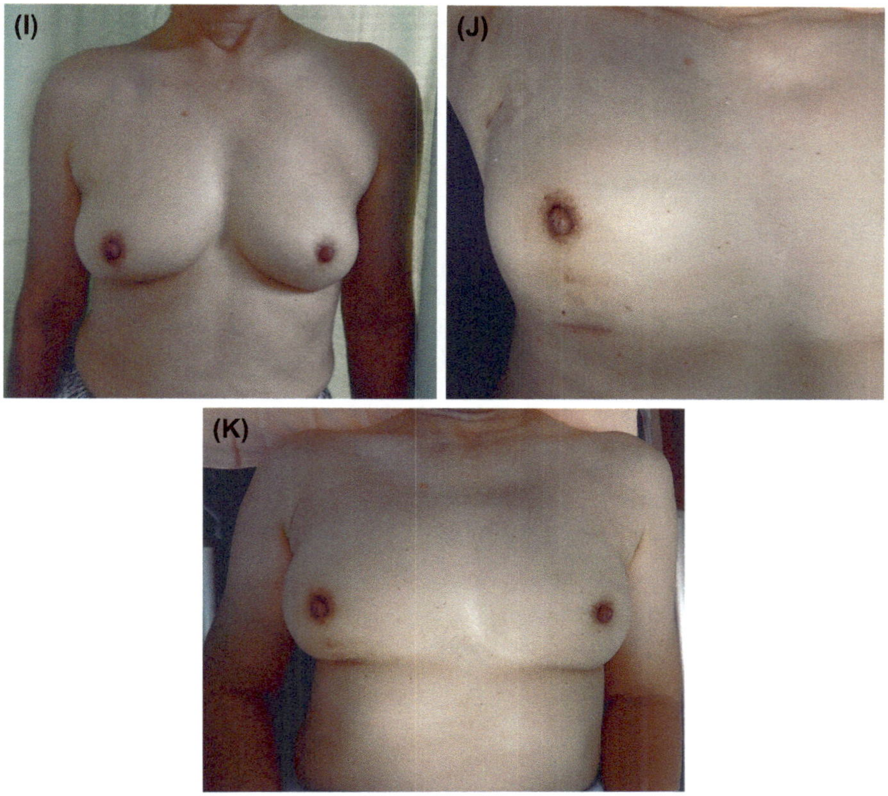

1.5I–K

1-month post-operative front and lateral views showing well-healed incisions that were barely visible.

Discussion

Endoscopic breast-conserving surgery offers a comparable alternative to conventional breast conservation techniques while providing better cosmesis with well-hidden, inconspicuous scars. Patient selection, however, still plays an important role in obtaining the maximal benefit from this technique (Ozaki & Ohara, 2014). Incision placement can be either single or dual incisions depending on tumour location (Nakajima et al., 2009; Tamaki et al., 2001). The two cases described in this chapter demonstrated the utilization of a single axillary incision for a tumour in the upper outer quadrant and a dual incision for a tumour located far from the nipple in the upper inner quadrant. In cases whereby the volume of resection is small to moderate, a level I oncoplastic procedure with volume displacement techniques suffice. Potential pitfalls with this technique may include inadequate resection margins as the endoscopic view lacks the tactile feedback in conventional surgery for palpable tumours. Hence, the authors advocate the use of intra-operative ultrasound for margin assessment as well as the utilization of blue dye in marking out the margins to act as a visual aid. In the authors' experience (Lai et al., 2017), endoscopic-assisted breast-conserving surgery has comparable short-term oncological safety profile to conventional breast-conserving surgery.

References

Lai, HW, Lin, HY, Chen, SL, Chen, ST, Chen, DR, Kuo, SJ, et al. (2017 Jan 11). Endoscopy-assisted surgery for the management of benign breast tumors: technique, learning curve, and patient-reported outcome from preliminary 323 procedures. *World J Surg Oncol, 15*(1), 19. https://doi.org/10.1186/s12957-016-1080-5. https://www.ncbi.nlm.nih.gov/pubmed/28077134. PMID:28077134.

Nakajima, H., Fujiwara, I., Mizuta, N., Sakaguchi, K., Hachimine, Y., & Magae, J. (2009). Video-assisted skin-sparing breast-conserving surgery for breast cancer and immediate reconstruction with autologous tissue: Clinical outcomes. *Annals of Surgical Oncology, 16*(7), 1982–1989. https://doi.org/10.1245/s10434-009-0429-1.

Ozaki, S., & Ohara, M. (2014). Endoscopy-assisted breast-conserving surgery for breast cancer patients. *Gland Surgery, 3*(2), 94–108. https://doi.org/10.3978/j.issn.2227-684X.2013.12.04.

Tamaki, Y., Sakita, I., Miyoshi, Y., Sekimoto, M., Takiguchi, S., Monden, M., et al. (2001). Transareolar endoscopy-assisted partial mastectomy: A preliminary report of six cases. *Surgical Laparoscopy, Endoscopy and Percutaneous Techniques*. https://doi.org/10.1097/00019509-200112000-00003.

CHAPTER 2

Endoscopic mastectomy

Description of technique

Pre-operative marking and positioning

Pre-operative marking was done with the patient in standing and supine position. After induction of general anaesthesia, the patient was then placed in supine position and ipsilateral arm abducted to 90 degrees to avoid affecting the operative procedure. Endoscopic video monitors (Olympus Optical Co., Tokyo, Japan) were set up on both sides of the patient's head to allow both the surgeon and assistant to view the monitor. An oblique-ended rigid endoscope measuring 5 mm in diameter with a viewing angle of 30 degrees was used in all procedures.

Axillary staging procedure

In patients for whom sentinel lymph node biopsy (SLNB) is indicated, a small amount (2−3 mCi) of radioisotope Tc99m was injected intradermally at the site of the tumour before operation (either on the day or 1 day prior).

After induction of general anaesthesia, 3 mL of 1% methylene blue (Merck, Darmstadt, Germany) was injected into the breast parenchyma in equally divided aliquots at five positions surrounding the hemisphere of the tumour facing the ipsilateral axilla. The breast tissue from the tumour to the axilla was then gently massaged for 5−10 minutes. Within 20−30 minutes after injection of the blue dye, a handheld gamma probe (Navigator; USSC, Norwalk, CT) was used to identify the hot spots, and the location of the hottest nodes was then marked. An approximately 3-cm oblique axillary incision was then made close to the hottest nodes, and SLNB was then performed. Fresh frozen section was performed as indicated. If SLN was positive for metastases, a complete axillary lymph node dissection up to level II was performed.

Dissection of breast parenchyma off pectoralis major fascia

The margin between pectoralis muscle and breast parenchyma was clearly identified. An endoscopic Ultra Retractor (Johnson & Johnson KK or Karl Storz) vein harvester was used for the dissection of pectoral muscle fascia off posterior portion of breast parenchyma. The penetrating vessels were coagulated and cut with bipolar

Minimally Invasive (Endoscopic & Robotic) Breast Surgery. https://doi.org/10.1016/B978-0-323-73405-9.00002-9

scissors (PowerStar, Johnson & Johnson KK) or a harmonic scalpel to ensure adequate haemostasis and therefore better visual clarity. Counter traction was applied by retracting surrounding tissue with the Ultra Retractor under endoscopic guidance to create a sufficient working space, and a suction tube can be used to evacuate mist and smoke.

Placement of single port, tunnelling, and development of skin flap (in cases of endoscopic mastectomy with insufflation technique)

To create a working space for placement of the single port (Glove Port; Nelis Corporation, Gyeonggi-do, Korea), a 3–4 cm subcutaneous flap was dissected with electrocautery under direct vision. Once adequate dissection was achieved, the single port was then inserted through the axilla incision and carbon dioxide (CO_2) insufflation with air pressure kept at 8 mmHg was used to create space for mastectomy. Dissection was then continued from the superficial skin flaps by dissecting the septa between the skin flap and parenchyma created by the tunnelling technique with monopolar scissors. A sub-areolar biopsy and fresh frozen section analysis can be performed in a nipple-sparing mastectomy. If cancer cell invasion was found in the sub-areolar area, the entire nipple-areolar complex (NAC) was removed and conversion to a skin-sparing mastectomy was then performed. After completion of the superficial skin flap dissection, dissection of the peripheral portion of the breast parenchyma was carried out subsequently. After completion of dissection, the entire breast specimen was removed through the axillary wound.

Tunnelling and development of skin flap (in cases of endoscopic mastectomy with retraction technique)

After completion of the axillary staging procedure, a semi-circular peri-areolar skin incision or a single axillary incision was made (depending on surgeon's preference) as previously described. A physiological saline solution containing lidocaine 0.05% and epinephrine 1:1,000,000 was injected subcutaneously into the whole breast to minimize bleeding. An approximately 3–5-mm-thick skin flap was created via tunnelling method using an optical bladeless trocar Xcel (Johnson & Johnson, Tokyo, Japan) under endoscopic guidance. Subsequently, the septa between the skin flap and parenchyma was dissected and taken off under endoscopic guidance using endoscissors, bipolar scissors, or a harmonic scalpel.

Mastectomy

At this stage of the operation, a gasless/retraction or insufflation technique can be employed, based on surgeon's preference. The authors used both techniques on a case-to-case basis and it will be shown in the case discussions. For insufflation technique, the authors preferred single port to multiple port sites, owing to better cosmesis.

After placement of a single port and CO_2 insufflation (for insufflation technique), the next step involved dissecting and taking off the septa between the skin flap and parenchyma under endoscopic guidance using endoscissors, monopolar or bipolar scissors, or a harmonic scalpel. Following adequate skin flap development, a sub-areolar biopsy and fresh frozen section analysis can be performed in a nipple-sparing mastectomy. If cancer cell invasion was found in the sub-areolar area, the entire NAC was removed and conversion to a skin-sparing mastectomy was then performed. After completion of skin flap development as well as detaching the breast off the pectoralis major fascia, the entire breast specimen can be removed via the axillary or peri-areolar incisions.

Case 6: endoscopic skin sparing mastectomy — dual incision, retraction technique

Patient/demographics

The patient is a 52-year-old lady with newly diagnosed clinical stage IIb (T2N1M0) left breast invasive ductal carcinoma, CerbB2+ in the retroareolar region. Her metastatic workup was negative. She underwent neoadjuvant chemotherapy and decided on a left nipple-sparing mastectomy without reconstruction. Even though her tumor did not show obvious extension to the nipple on her breast magnetic resonance imaging (MRI), she was counseled regarding intra-op sub-nipple frozen section analysis and the risks of involvement would then warrant excision of nipple—areolar complex (NAC) in which she was agreeable.

Surgery and pathology report

The patient underwent endoscopic nipple-sparing mastectomy with sentinel lymph node biopsy without reconstruction. The patient had a dual incision in view of location of tumor, and the frozen section of sub-nipple tissue biopsy showed tumor involvement. Conversion to skin-sparing mastectomy was then performed. Sentinel lymph node biopsy was negative. Final histopathology revealed residual 3 mm IDC (ypT1aN0M0).

Post-operative outcomes

There were no immediate post-operative complications, and the patient was discharged well. In addition, she was reviewed in the outpatient clinic with satisfactory reporting of her cosmetic outcomes. She did not undergo further adjuvant therapy as she was not keen.

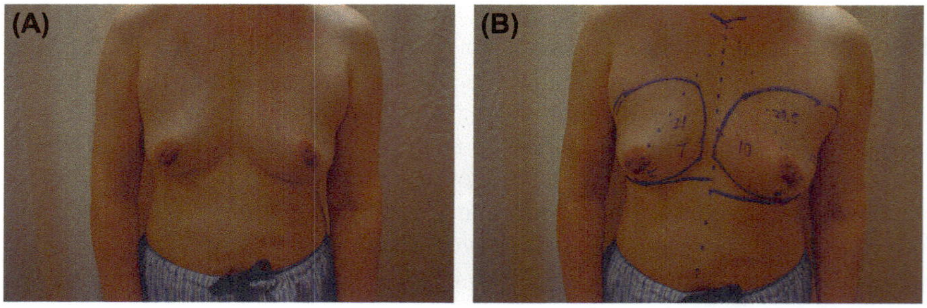

2.6A, B

Pre-operative front views showing pre-operative markings.

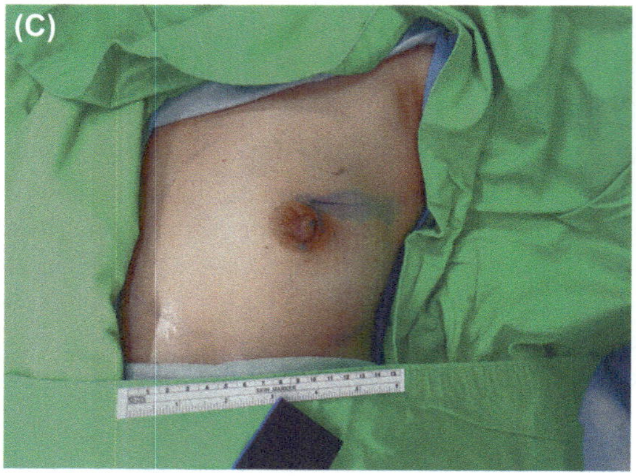

2.6C

On-table view after injection of methylene blue dye in the periareolar region.

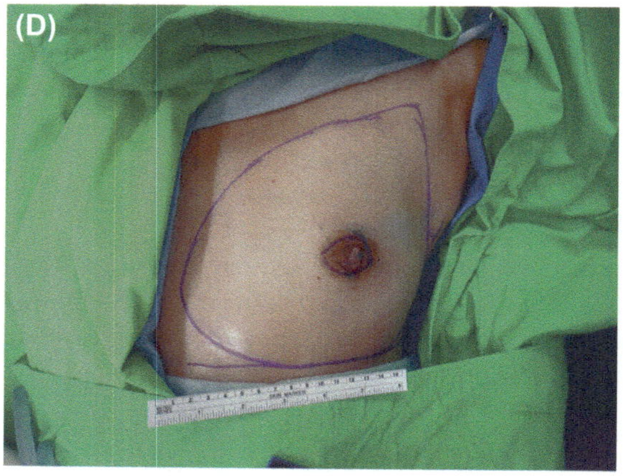

2.6D

Markings showing the breast footprint and extent of dissection.

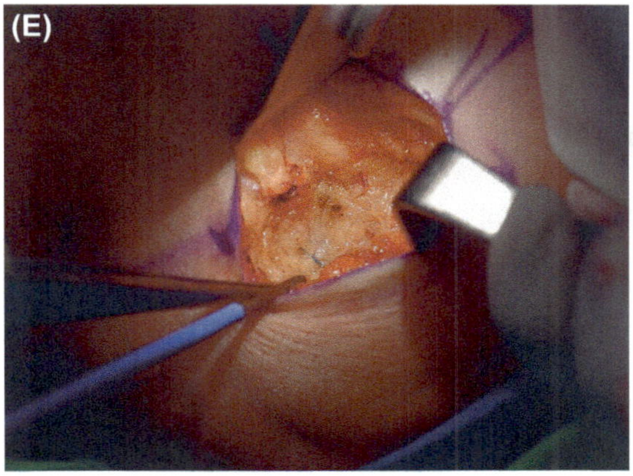

2.6E

Sentinel lymph node visualized.

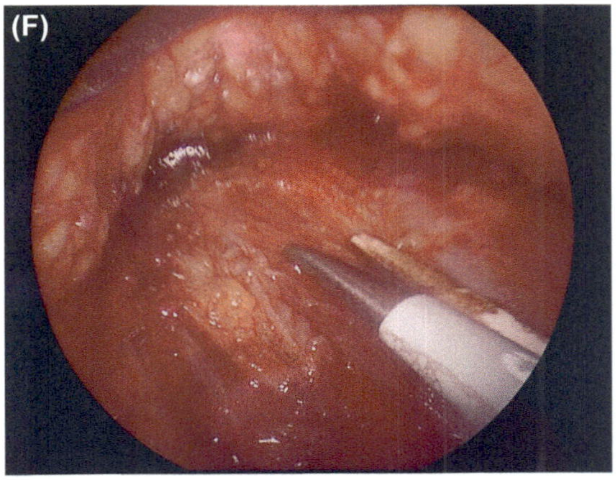

2.6F

Endoscopic Ultra Retractor (Johnson & Johnson KK or Karl Storz) vein harvester used for the dissection of pectoral muscle fascia off posterior portion of breast parenchyma.

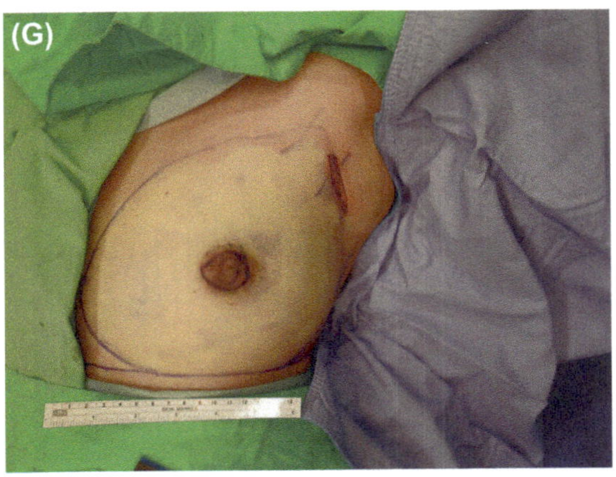

2.6G

Axillary incision shown here after completion of sentinel lymph node biopsy.

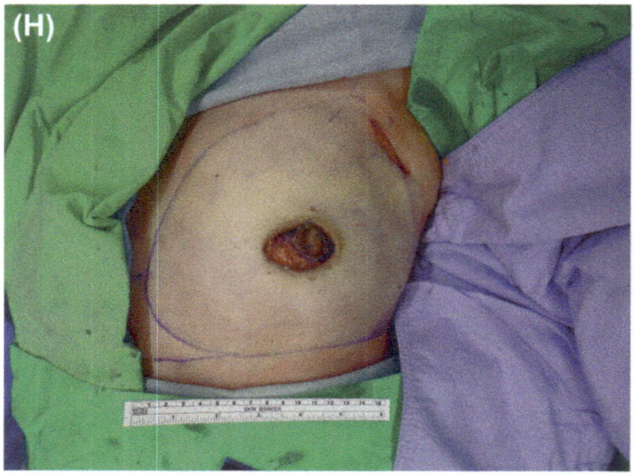

2.6H

A second peri-areolar incision used in view of tumor location.

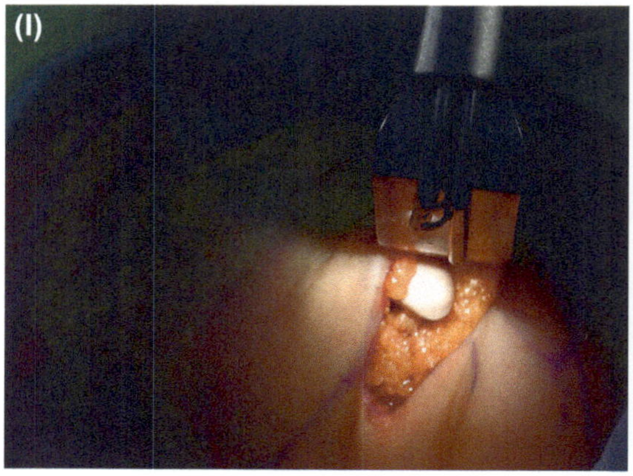

2.6I

Both incisions were connected as shown in this picture.

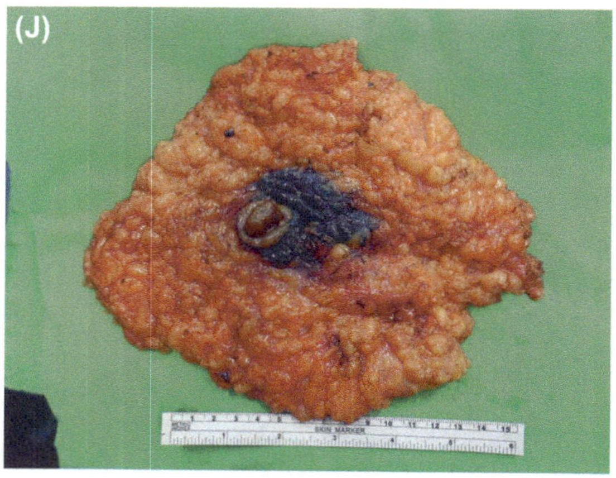

2.6J

Mastectomy specimen removed intact.

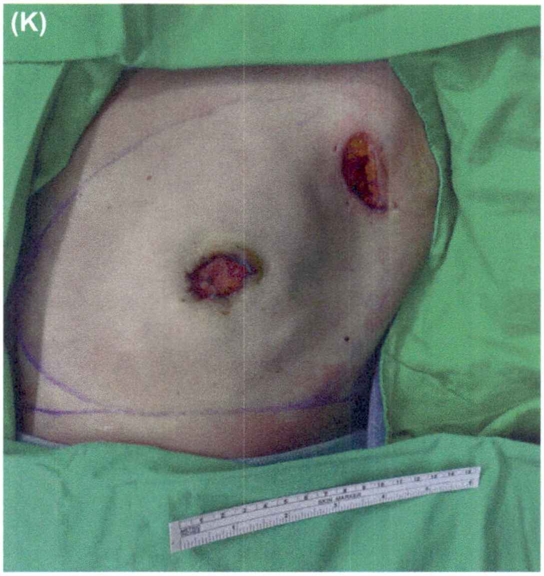

2.6K

Immediate post-operative front view showing both incisions and removal of NAC due to positive frozen section.

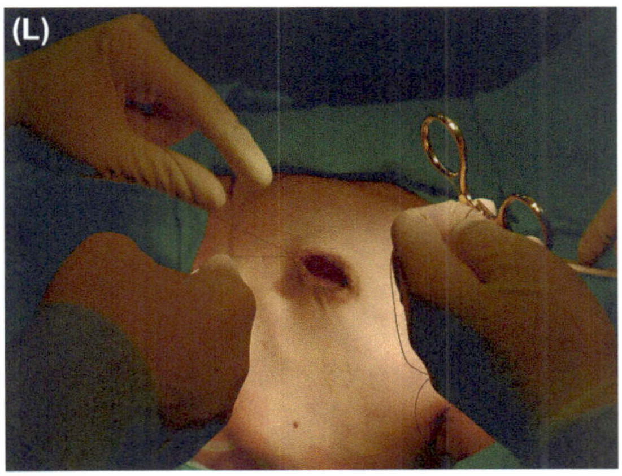

2.6L

Closure of nipple incision using purse-string technique.

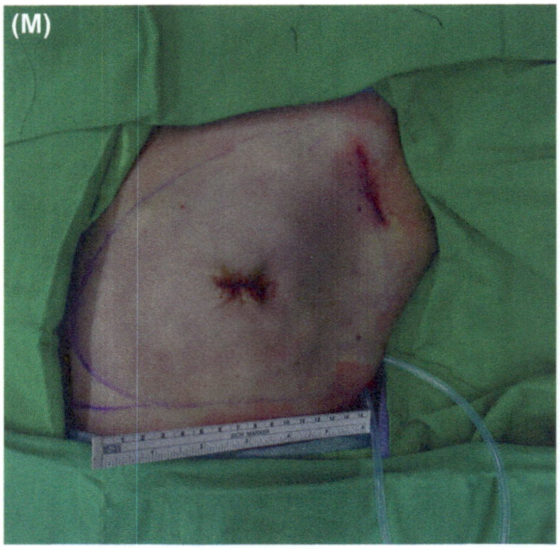

2.6M

Final immediate post-operative front view.

Case 7: endoscopic nipple-sparing mastectomy – single incision, insufflation technique

Patient/demographics

The case described a 55-year-old lady diagnosed with clinical stage IIb left breast invasive ductal carcinoma.

Her metastatic workup did not reveal any distant metastases.

This lady received neoadjuvant chemotherapy followed with a left nipple-sparing mastectomy with no reconstruction thereafter.

Surgery and pathology report

The patient underwent left endoscopic nipple-sparing mastectomy with sentinel lymph node biopsy. Sentinel lymph node biopsy did not reveal any metastasis. Intra-operative frozen section for sub-nipple biopsy was negative. Her final histology revealed residual DCIS (ypTisN0M0).

Post-operative outcomes

There were no immediate complications, and the patient was discharged well 2 days after operation. The patient did not receive any adjuvant therapy thereafter.

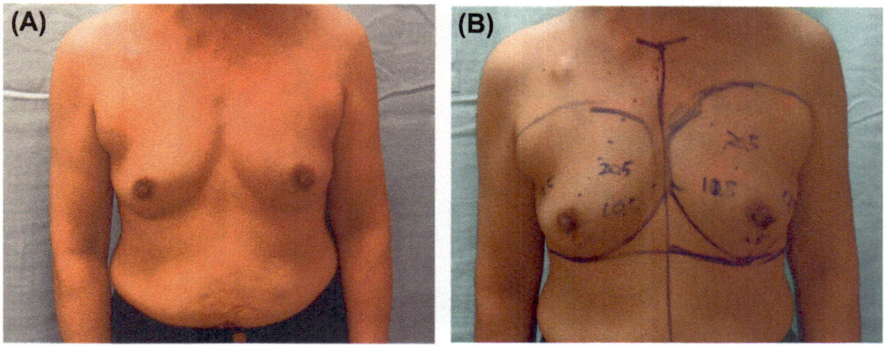

2.7A, B

Pre-operative front views showing operative markings. Chemotherapy port was also seen in the right infraclavicular region.

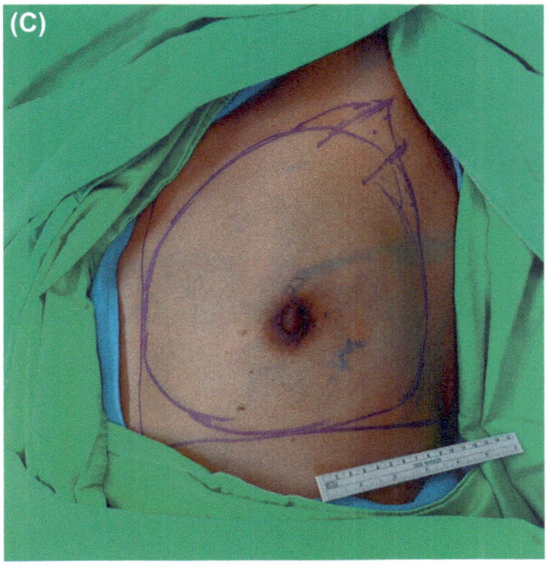

2.7C

On-table view after injection of methylene blue dye in the periareolar region. Markings showing the breast footprint and extent of dissection.

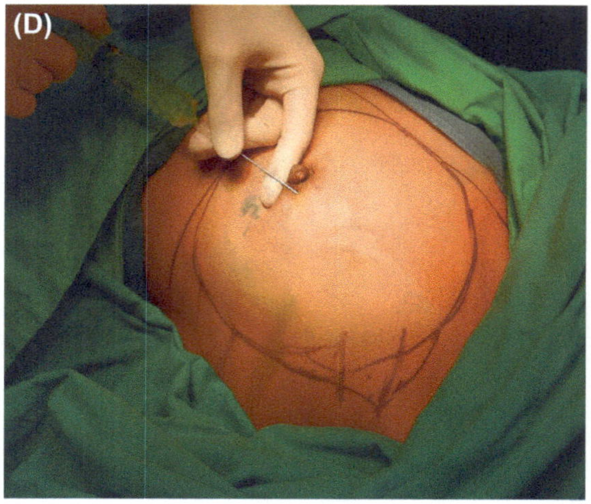

2.7D

Infiltration of tumescent solution to aid in plane dissection and haemostasis.

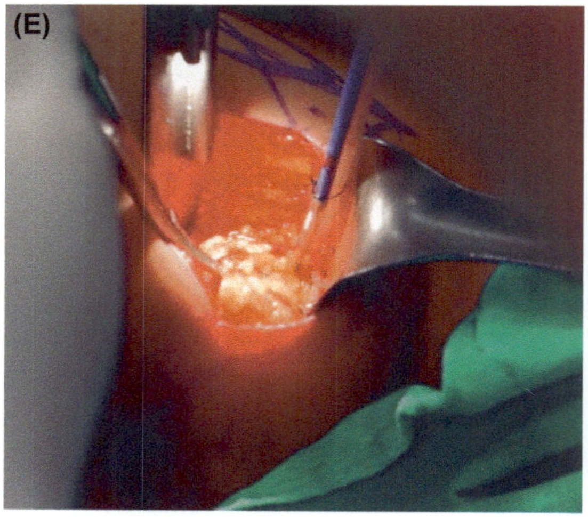

2.7E

Sentinel lymph node biopsy performed under direct vision.

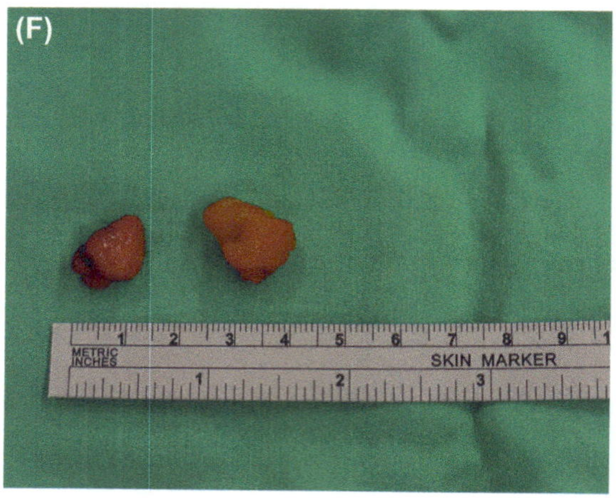

2.7F

Sentinel lymph nodes identified with dual modality.

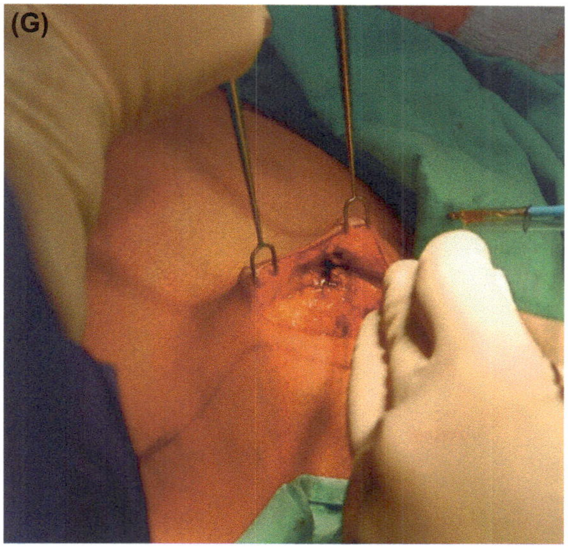

2.7G

Creation of working space for placement of single port.

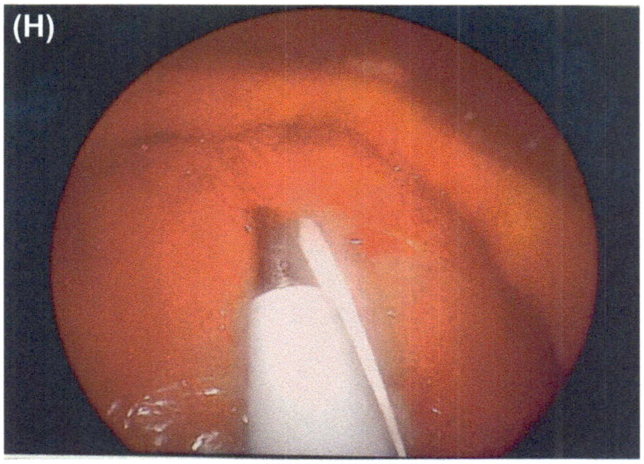

2.7H

Endoscopic Ultra Retractor (Johnson & Johnson KK or Karl Storz) vein harvester used for the dissection of pectoral muscle fascia off posterior portion of breast parenchyma.

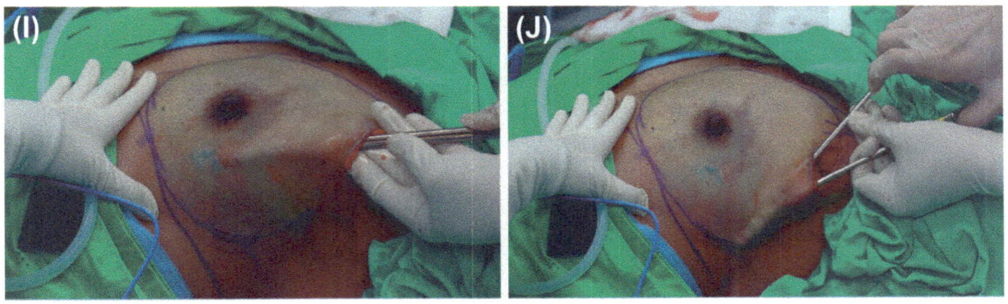

2.7I, J

Tunneling technique with blunt dissection using scissors.

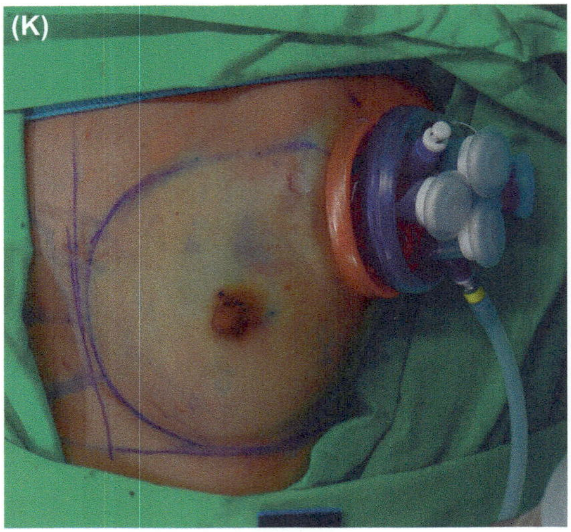

2.7K

Placement of the single port (Glove Port; Nelis Corporation, Gyeonggi-do, Korea) before commencement of mastectomy.

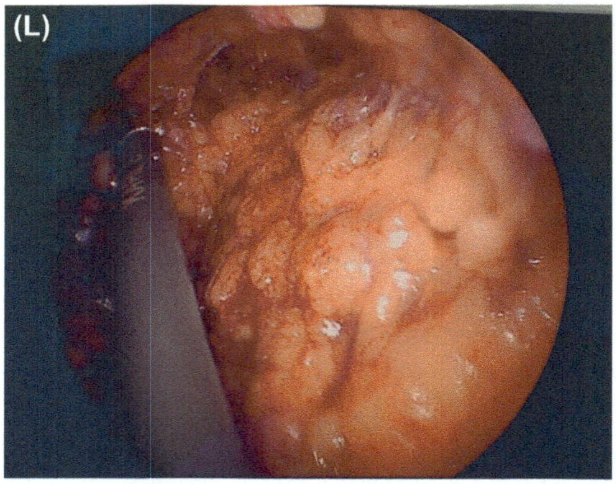

2.7L

Endoscopic view showing dissection of septa between skin flap and breast parenchyma.

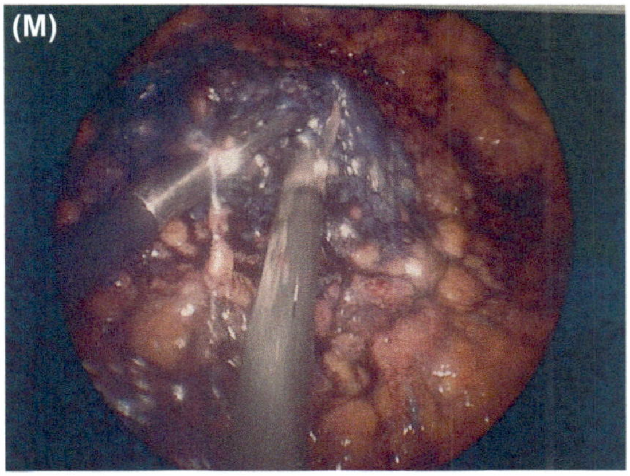

2.7M

Endoscopic view showing sub-nipple biopsy taken for intra-operative frozen section.

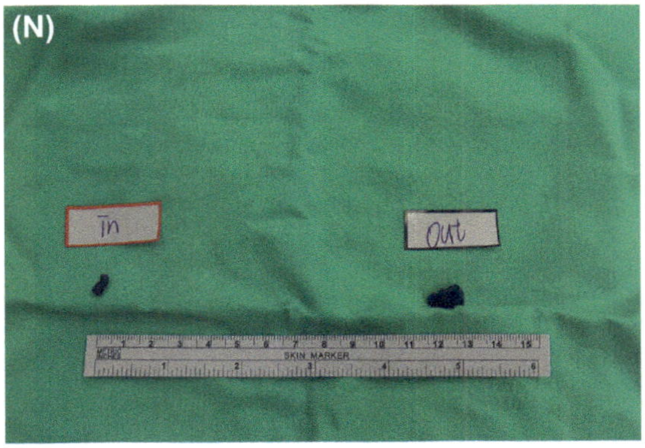

2.7N

Sub-nipple biopsy sent off as inner and outer region to reduce false negative.

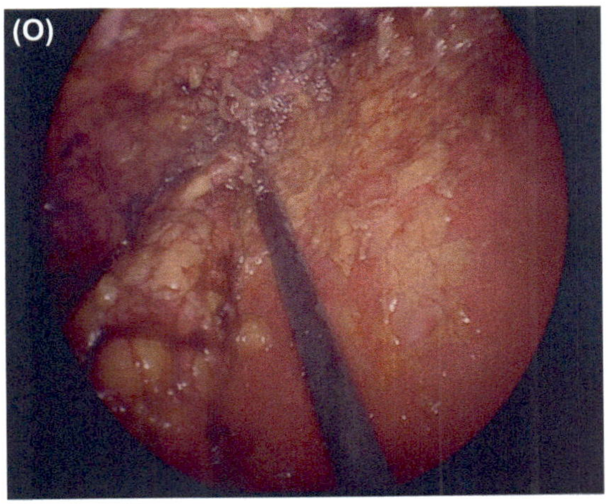

2.7O

Endoscopic view showing dissection of breast parenchyma nearing completion of mastectomy.

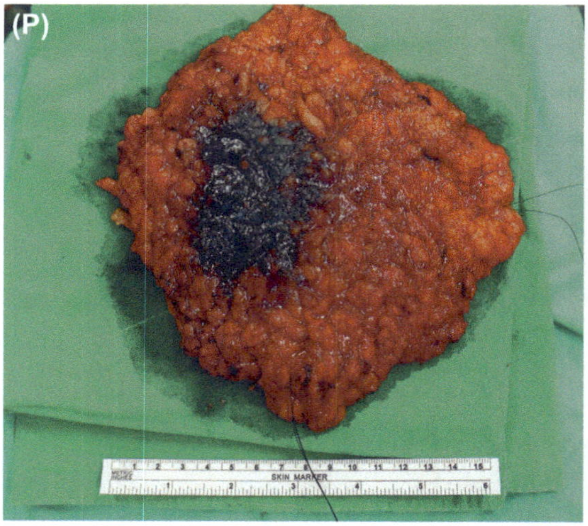

2.7P

Mastectomy specimen removed intact.

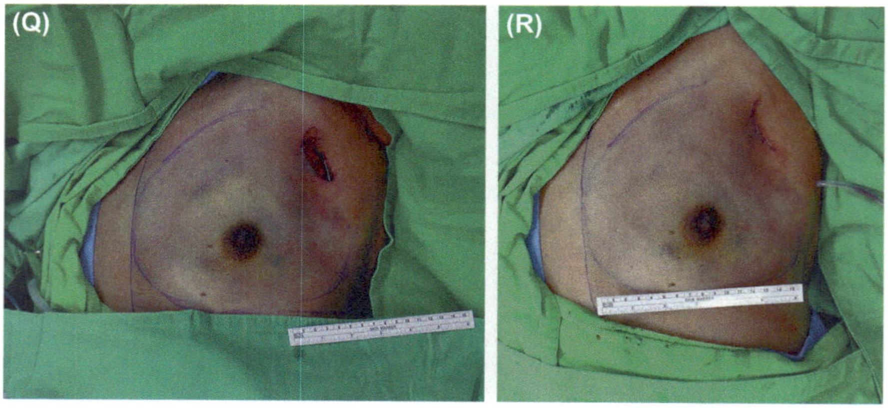

2.7Q, R

Immediate post-operative views showing single axillary incision.

Case 8: endoscopic nipple-sparing mastectomy – bilateral, single incision, insufflation technique with 3D endoscope

Patient/demographics

The case described a 53-year-old lady diagnosed with clinical stage IIb left breast triple negative invasive ductal carcinoma who underwent neoadjuvant chemotherapy with complete radiological response. Her metastatic workup did not reveal any distant metastases. The patient opted for a nipple-sparing mastectomy along with risk-reducing mastectomy on the contralateral side with no reconstruction.

Surgery and pathology report

The patient underwent bilateral endoscopic nipple-sparing mastectomy with left sentinel lymph node biopsy using three-dimensional (3D) endoscopic system (KARL STORZ, Germany). Sentinel lymph node biopsy did not reveal any metastasis. Intra-operative frozen section for sub-nipple biopsy was negative on both sides. Her final histology revealed residual DCIS (ypTisN0M0), whereas the contralateral breast showed no evidence of abnormalities.

Post-operative outcomes

There were no immediate complications, and the patient was discharged well 4 days after operation. The patient did not receive any adjuvant therapy thereafter.

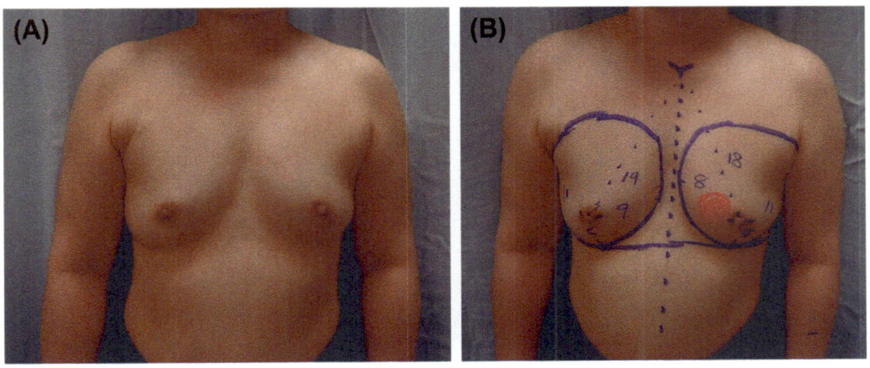

2.8A, B

Pre-operative front views of the patient.

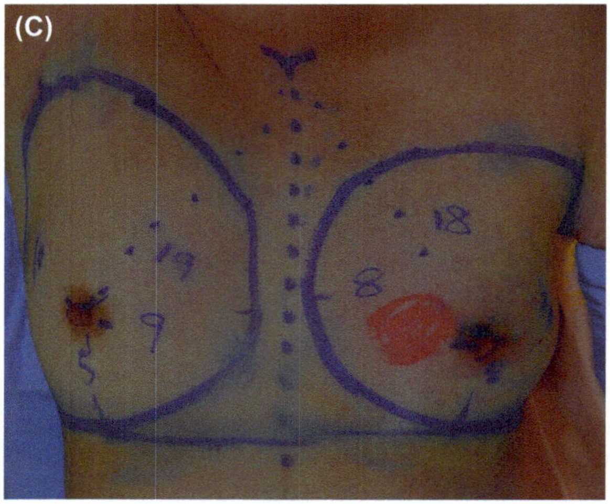

2.8C

On-table view demonstrating pre-operative markings as well as tumor location (note: patient had complete radiological response, and marking was used to illustrate location of primary tumor).

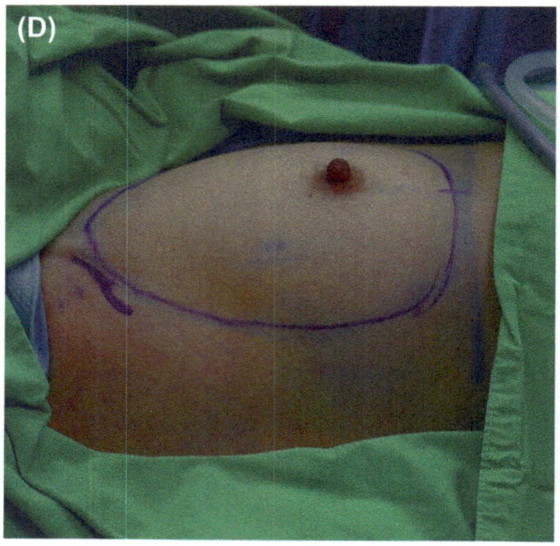

2.8D

On-table view showing axillary incision planned for the right side.

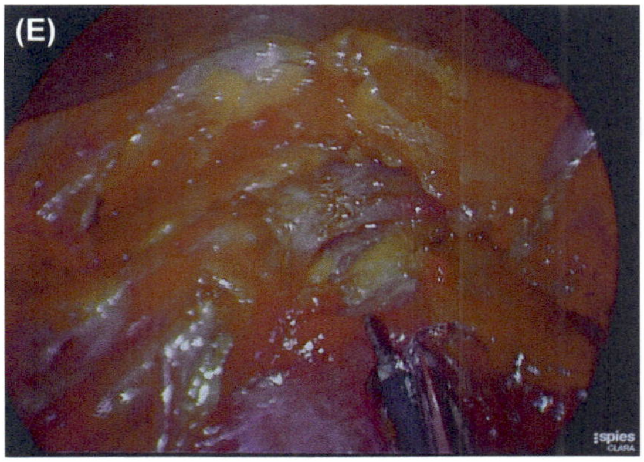

2.8E

Endoscopic Ultra Retractor (Johnson & Johnson KK or Karl Storz) vein harvester used for the dissection of pectoral muscle fascia off posterior portion of breast parenchyma.

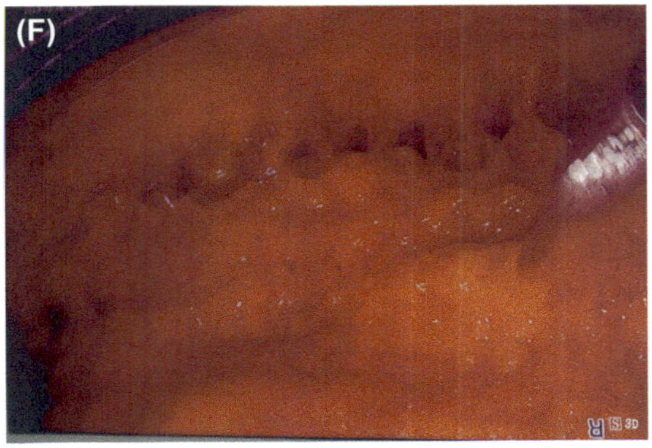

2.8F

Endoscopic view on the monitor (without 3D glasses).

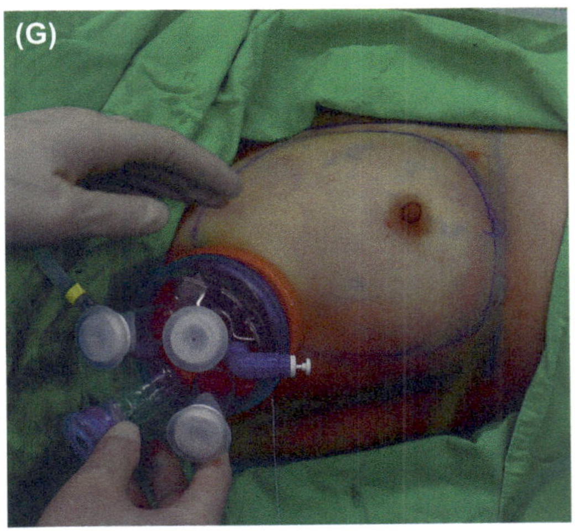

2.8G

Placement of the single port (Glove Port; Nelis Corporation, Gyeonggi-do, Korea) before commencement of mastectomy.

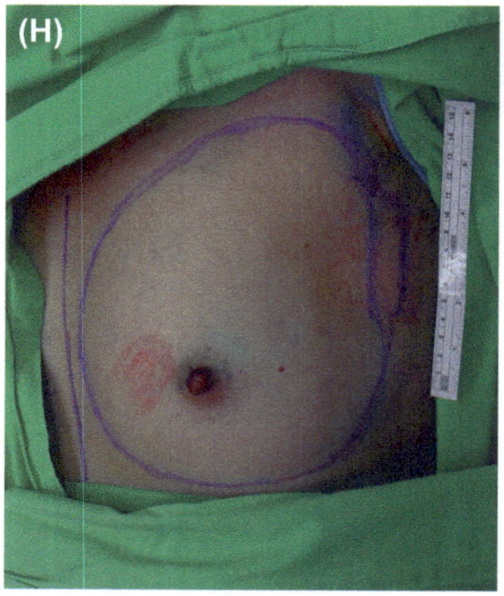

2.8H

On-table view showing pre-operative marking with incision planned along anterior axillary line (note: incision over right side was placed over the axilla as patient had a right accessory breast tissue excision performed before).

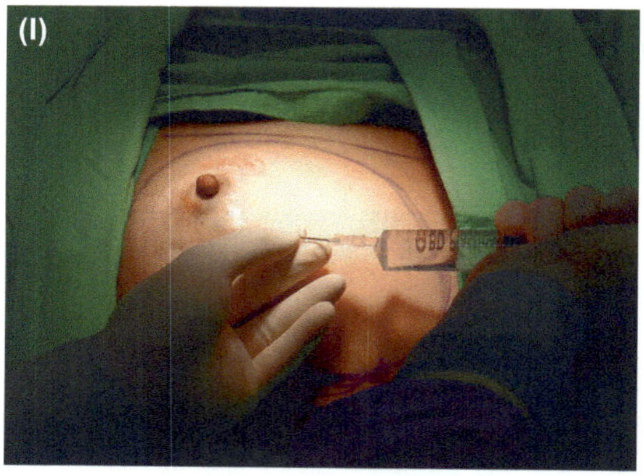

2.8I

Infiltration of tumescent solution to aid in plane dissection and haemostasis.

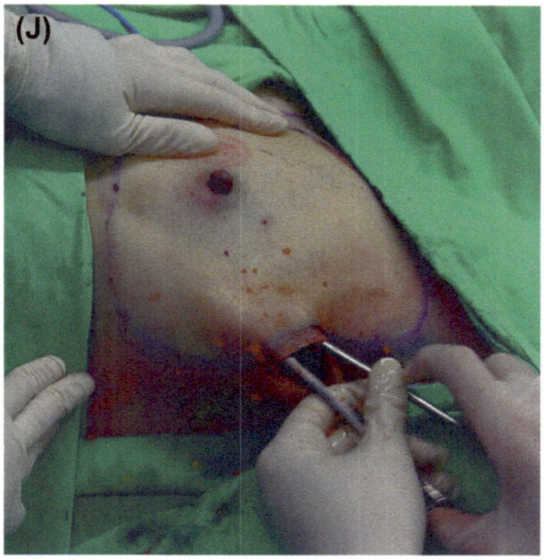

2.8J

Tunneling technique with blunt dissection using scissors.

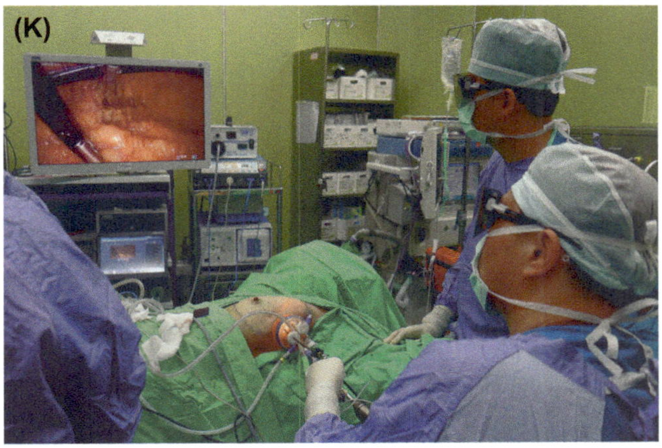

2.8K

Intra-operative layout demonstration of the position of surgeon, first assistant, and patient in relation to the endoscopic system.

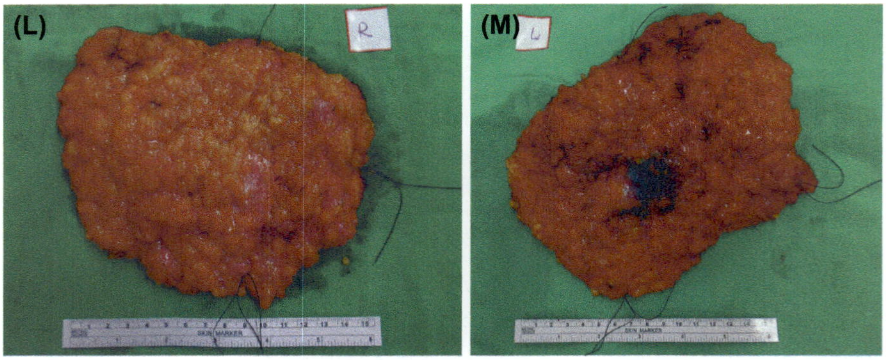

2.8L, M

Bilateral mastectomy specimens removed intact and oriented with silk sutures.

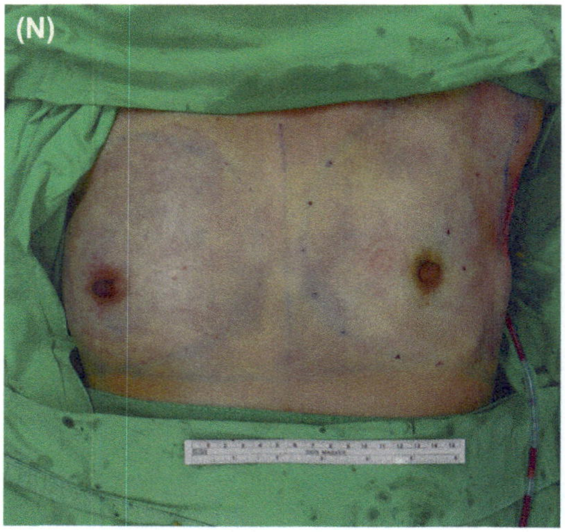

2.8N

Immediate post-operative view showing well-hidden incisions.

Discussion

Endoscopic nipple-sparing mastectomy can be offered to patients who are not keen for reconstruction after mastectomy but keen to preserve their nipple-areolar complex (NAC). Patients, however, need to be counselled for the possibility of conversion to a skin-sparing mastectomy should intra-operative frozen section demonstrate any involvement. In Case 6 described at the start of this chapter, the NAC was removed as intra-operative frozen section showed involvement and the wound was subsequently closed in purse-string fashion. In addition, patient will have to be advised regarding the asymmetry expected with no reconstruction performed. From the authors' experience (Lai et al., 2016, 2015), a significant number of patients who underwent this procedure were satisfied with the cosmesis but most importantly, most patients were glad to preserve the NAC and felt that was more significant than asymmetry or cosmesis. With regards to the choice of incision, endoscopic nipple-sparing mastectomy can be performed with either a single incision or dual incision (axillary and peri-areolar) (Lai et al., 2018). It will eventually goes down to tumour location as well as surgeon's preference. Technical variations also include the use of insufflation or retraction in the conduct of the operation. The advantage with insufflation technique will mainly be better visualization and working space in which retraction technique is lacking; whereas, the disadvantage will be fogging of the lens and view which is normally less with retraction technique. Potential pitfalls with this technique may include uneven skin flap due to lack of tactile feedback, but this could potentially be avoided after overcoming the initial learning curve. The authors would also suggest to use bimanual palpation while developing skin flap to reduce the risk of skin flap being raised too thin.

References

Lai, H. W., Chen, S. T., Chen, D. R., Chen, S. L., Chang, T. W., Kuo, S. J., et al. (2016). Current trends in and indications for endoscopy-assisted breast surgery for breast cancer: Results from a six-year study conducted by the taiwan endoscopic breast surgery cooperative group. *PLoS One*. https://doi.org/10.1371/journal.pone.0150310.

Lai, H. W., Lin, S. L., Chen, S. T., Kuok, K. M., Chen, S. L., Lin, Y. L., et al. (2018). Single-axillary-incision endoscopic-assisted hybrid technique for nipple-sparing mastectomy: Technique, preliminary results, and patient-reported cosmetic outcome from preliminary 50 procedures. *Annals of Surgical Oncology, 25*(5), 1340–1349. https://doi.org/10.1245/s10434-018-6383-z.

Lai, H. W., Wu, H. S., Chuang, K. L., Chen, D. R., Chang, T. W., Kuo, S. J., et al. (2015). Endoscopy-assisted total mastectomy followed by immediate pedicled transverse rectus abdominis musculocutaneous (TRAM) flap reconstruction: Preliminary results of 48 patients. *Surgical Innovation*. https://doi.org/10.1177/1553350614546003.

SECTION

2

Endoscopic breast conserving surgery with immediate reconstruction

CHAPTER

3

Endoscopic breast-conserving surgery with immediate omental flap reconstruction

Description of technique

Pre-operative marking and positioning

Pre-operative marking was done with the patient in standing and supine position. After induction of general anaesthesia, the patient was then placed in the supine position and ipsilateral arm abducted to 90 degrees to avoid affecting the operative procedure. Endoscopic video monitors (Olympus Optical Co., Tokyo, Japan) were set up on both sides of the patient's head to allow both the surgeon and the assistant to view the monitor. An oblique-ended rigid endoscope measuring 5 mm in diameter with a viewing angle of 30 degrees was used in all procedures.

Axillary staging procedure

In patients for whom sentinel lymph node biopsy (SLNB) is indicated, a small amount (2–3 mCi) of radioisotope Tc99m was injected intradermally at the site of the tumour before operation (either on the day or 1 day prior).

After induction of general anaesthesia, 3 mL of 1% methylene blue (Merck, Darmstadt, Germany) was injected into the breast parenchyma in equally divided aliquots at five positions surrounding the hemisphere of the tumour facing the ipsilateral axilla. The breast tissue from the tumour to the axilla was then gently massaged for 5–10 minutes. Within 20–30 minutes after injection of the blue dye, a handheld gamma probe (Navigator; USSC, Norwalk, CT) was used to identify the hot spots, and the location of the hottest nodes was then marked. An approximately 3-cm oblique axillary incision was then made close to the hottest nodes, and SLNB was then performed. Fresh frozen section was performed as indicated. If SLN was positive for metastases, a complete axillary lymph node dissection up to level II was performed.

Dissection of breast parenchyma off pectoralis major fascia

After completion of axillary staging procedure, dissection was carried out to the lateral border of the pectoralis major muscle. The margin between pectoralis

Minimally Invasive (Endoscopic & Robotic) Breast Surgery. https://doi.org/10.1016/B978-0-323-73405-9.00003-0

muscle and breast parenchyma was clearly identified. An endoscopic Ultra Retractor (Johnson & Johnson KK or Karl Storz) vein harvester was used for the dissection pectoral muscle fascia off posterior portion of breast parenchyma. The penetrating vessels were coagulated and cut with bipolar scissors (PowerStar, Johnson & Johnson KK) or a harmonic scalpel to ensure adequate haemostasis and therefore better visual clarity. Counter traction was applied by retracting surrounding tissue with the Ultra Retractor under endoscopic guidance to create a sufficient working space, and a suction tube can be used to evacuate mist and smoke.

Tunnelling and development of skin flap

After completion of the axillary staging procedure, a semi-circular peri-areolar skin incision or an inframammary crease incision was made (depending on tumour location or surgeon's preference). A physiological saline solution containing lidocaine 0.05% and epinephrine 1:1,000,000 was injected subcutaneously into the whole breast to minimize bleeding. An approximately 3–5-mm-thick skin flap was created via tunnelling method using an optical bladeless trocar Xcel (Johnson & Johnson, Tokyo, Japan) under endoscopic guidance. Subsequently, the septa between the skin flap and parenchyma was dissected and taken off under endoscopic guidance using endoscissors, bipolar scissors, or a harmonic scalpel.

Performing wide excision and repair of resection cavity

After development of adequate skin flap (either via a single axillary or combination of axillary and peri-areolar or inframammary incision), wide excision was performed using bipolar or monopolar diathermy. To guide resection with adequate margins, the authors recommended the use of intra-operative ultrasound and marking of resection margin with blue dye injection. Specimen was retrieved thereafter and haemostasis secured.

Laparoscopic pedicled omental flap harvest and reconstruction

With the patient placed in the supine position, a 10-mm camera port was placed through an infraumbilical incision via open cutdown. Pneumoperitoneum was then created with CO_2 insufflation. Three working ports were then placed with two over the right lumbar region (both 5 mm) and one over the left (12 mm). After gross inspection of the intra-abdominal cavity to ensure no abnormalities seen, omentum was identified and lifted up. Dissection of the omentum was performed slightly left to the centre of the transverse colon and advanced towards the splenic flexure using a harmonic scalpel (Ethicon Ecdo-Surgery Inc., Cincinnati, OH). Care must be taken to ligate and divide the left gastroepiploic vessels near the spleen. All other branches were divided as close to the stomach as possible. In a pedicled omental flap, the right gastroepiploic vessels were preserved as the feeding vessels for the flap and the dissection should stop right past the pyloric channel, after confirming preservation of the right gastroepiploic vessels. After isolation of the flap was completed, an approximately 2–3-finger breadths subcutaneous tunnel was prepared from the medial end of the inframammary fold (a new incision may be required if not through the same incision for wide excision) towards the xiphoid process till the linea alba was encountered. Thereafter, a 2–3 cm longitudinal incision was made on the linea alba and abdominal cavity entered to deliver the flap. Care must be taken to avoid twisting of pedicle. Securing the flap to the resection cavity with absorbable sutures was then performed at the end of the reconstruction. Drain was placed on a case-to-case basis or based on the surgeon's preference.

Case 9: endoscopic breast-conserving surgery with immediate pedicled omental flap reconstruction – inframammary crease incision

Patient/demographics

This is a case of a 40-year-old lady with a 2-cm tumor in the lower inner quadrant of the right breast. Core biopsy pre-operatively revealed an invasive ductal carcinoma, ER/PR+, CerbB2+.

Her metastatic workup was negative. The patient was keen to undergo breast conservation with reconstruction. In view of favourable tumor location, she was offered a partial reconstruction with a pedicled omental flap.

Surgery and pathology report

The patient underwent endoscopic breast-conserving surgery with sentinel lymph node biopsy and immediate laparoscopic pedicled omental flap reconstruction. Sentinel lymph node biopsy was negative for metastases. Her final histology showed a stage I disease (T1cN0M0), and the patient subsequently received adjuvant radiotherapy and endocrine therapy for 5 years.

Post-operative outcomes

No immediate complications were encountered, and the patient was discharged 2 days after operation. She was reviewed in the outpatient clinic and reported satisfactory cosmesis at her 1-month follow-up.

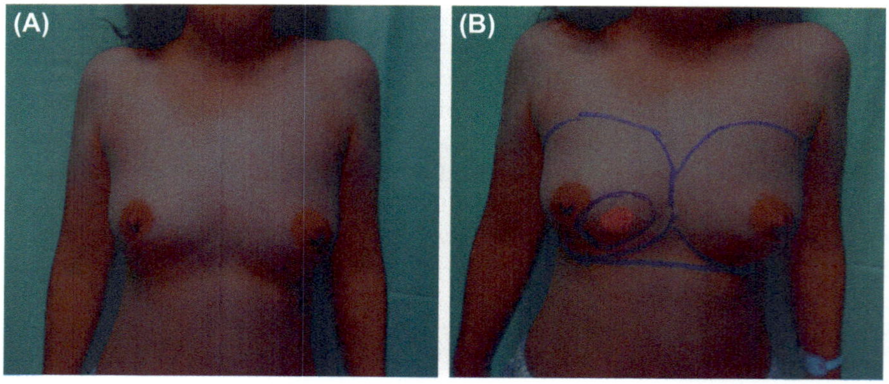

3.9A, B

Pre-operative front views showing pre-operative markings and location of tumor.

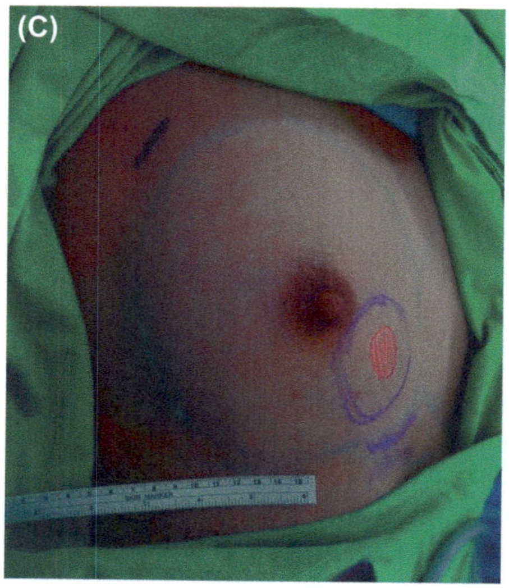

3.9C

On-table view with markings of planned incisions seen here.

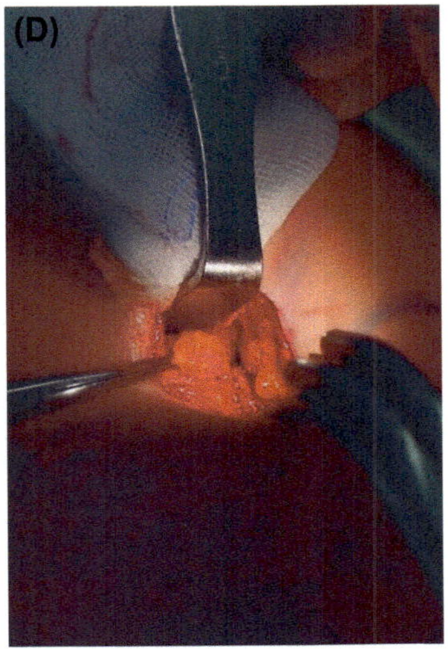

3.9D

Sentinel lymph node biopsy identified as shown here.

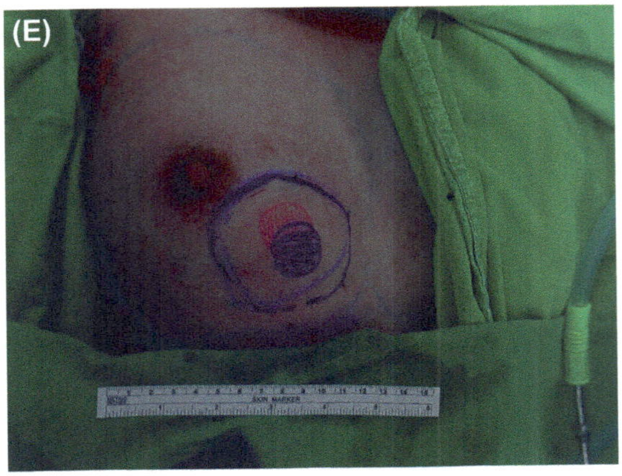

3.9E

Completion of sentinel lymph node biopsy and inframammary incision planned for both wide excision and access to pedicle omental flap.

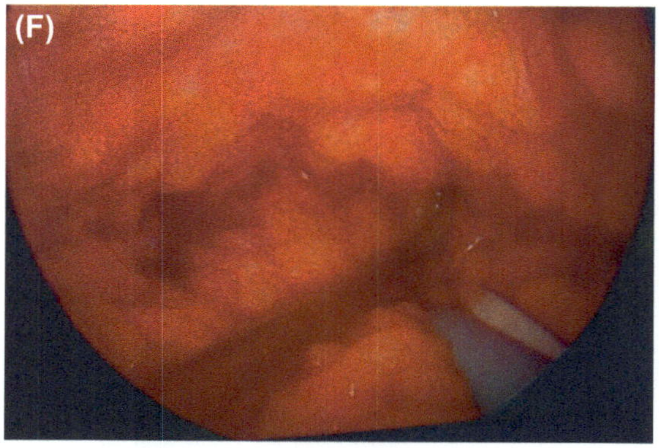

3.9F

Endoscopic view showing raising of skin flap and dissection of septa between skin and breast parenchyma.

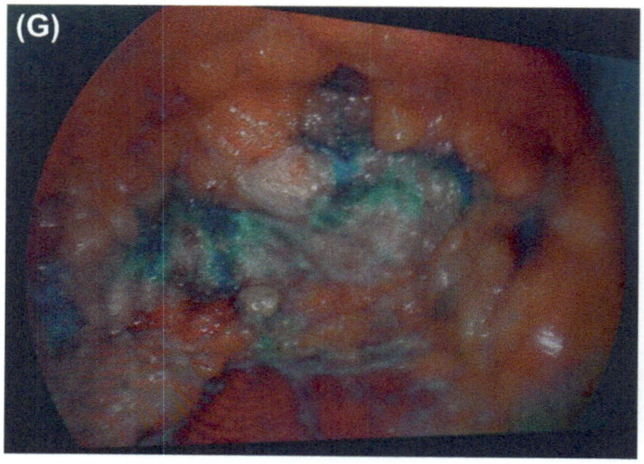

3.9G

Endoscopic view showing the cavity after wide excision.

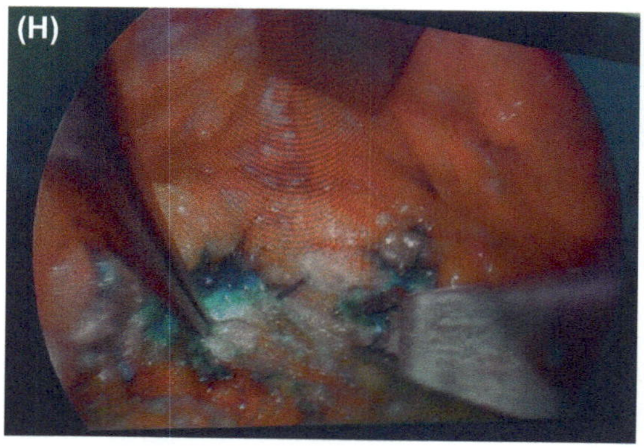

3.9H

Endoscopic view showing placement of marker clip along margins of resection cavity.

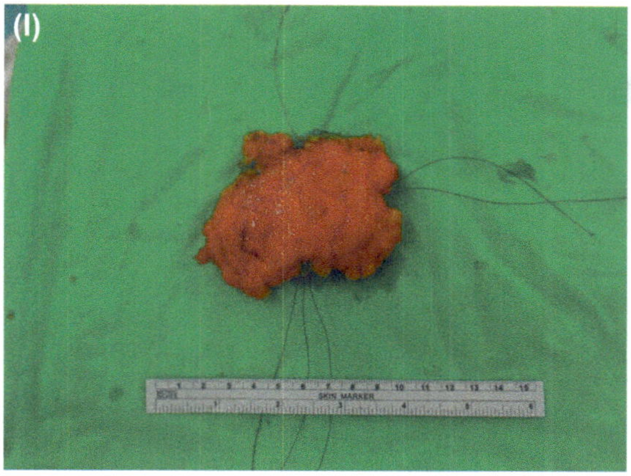

3.9I

Wide excision specimen removed intact.

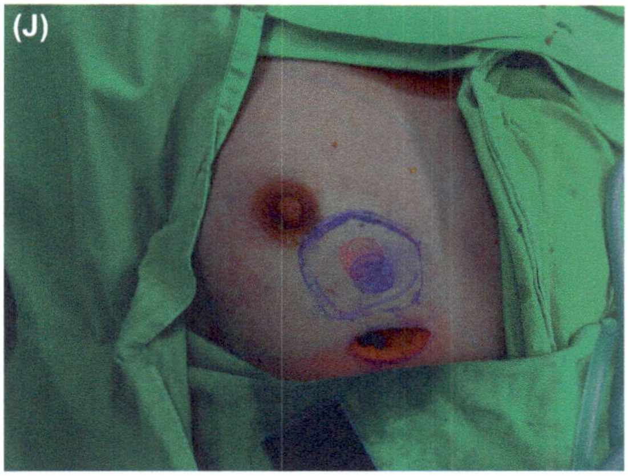

3.9J

Immediate view post wide excision.

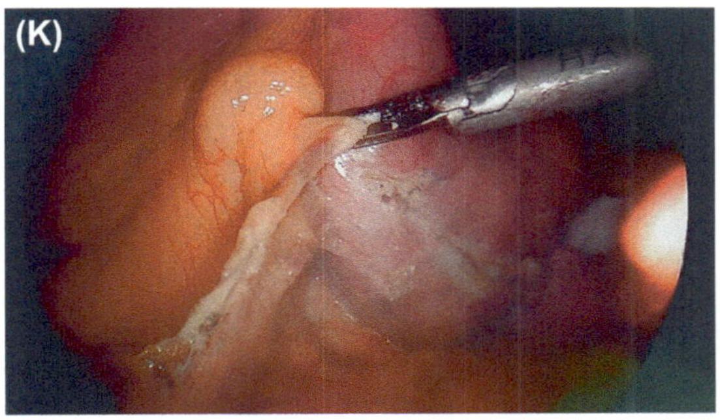

3.9K

Endoscopic view showing the harvest of omental flap, and greater omentum was taken close to the stomach with preservation of the right gastroepiploic vessels as the feeding vessels for the flap.

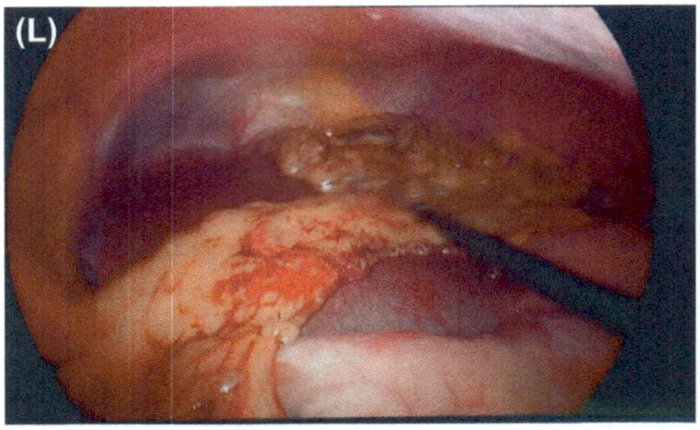

3.9L

Flap completely raised and ready to be exteriorized via an incision over linea alba.

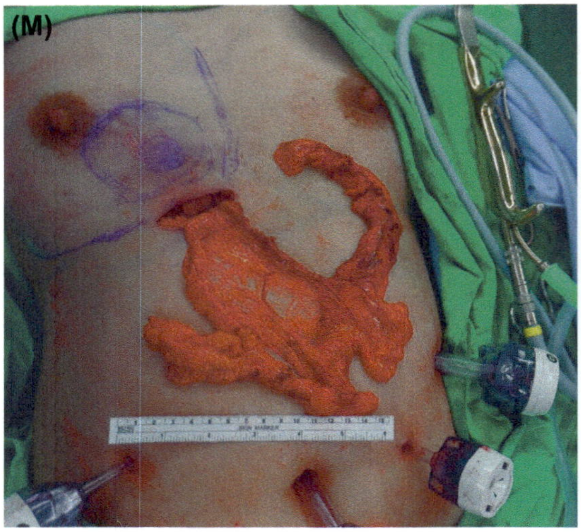

3.9M

Flap exteriorized and subsequently anchored to the resection cavity bed.

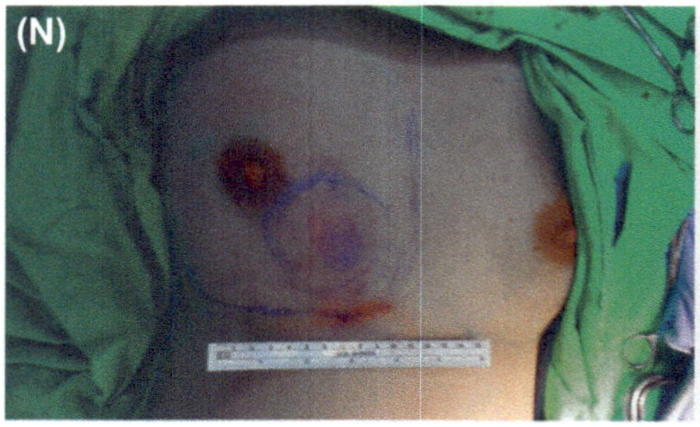

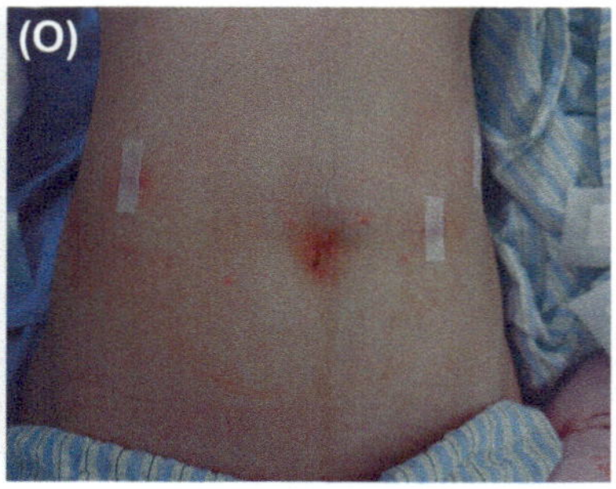

3.9N, O

Immediate post-operative views showing incisions that were small and well hidden.

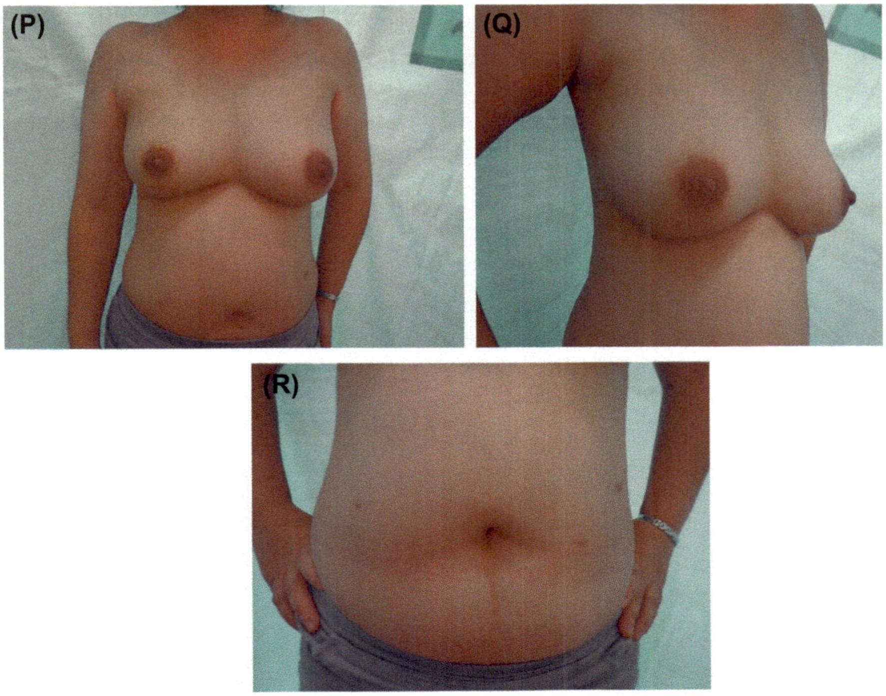

3.9P–R

1-month post-operative views showing well-healed and well-hidden scars providing excellent cosmesis for both donor and wide excision sites.

Case 10: endoscopic breast-conserving surgery with immediate pedicled omental flap reconstruction – inframammary crease incision

Patient/demographics

The case described a 41-year-old lady diagnosed with clinical stage I left breast cancer with a pre-operative core biopsy report of an invasive ductal carcinoma ER/PR +, CerbB2 equivocal.

Her metastatic workup did not reveal any distant metastases.

The patient was keen for breast conservation with partial reconstruction.

Clinically, the tumor was adherent to the overlying skin but there was no ulceration. The patient was advised to remove skin overlying the tumor to which she agreed.

She decided for an endoscopic breast-conserving surgery with pedicled omental flap reconstruction.

Surgery and pathology report

The patient underwent endoscopic breast-conserving surgery with sentinel lymph node biopsy and immediate pedicled omental flap reconstruction. Sentinel lymph node biopsy returned negative. Her final pathology report returned as a stage I (T1cN0M0) disease and patient subsequently received post-operative radiotherapy and endocrine therapy for 5 years.

Post-operative outcomes

Patient was discharged 2 days after operation with no immediate complications encountered. She was reviewed in clinic twice a week and a review 2 weeks after her operation showed satisfactory cosmesis.

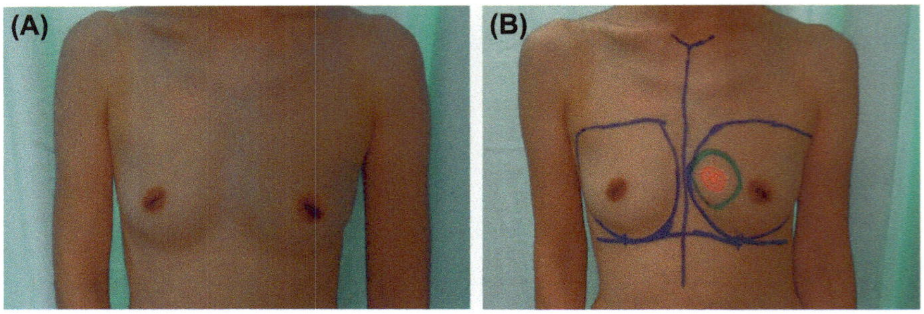

3.10A, B

Pre-operative front views showing pre-operative markings and location of tumor.

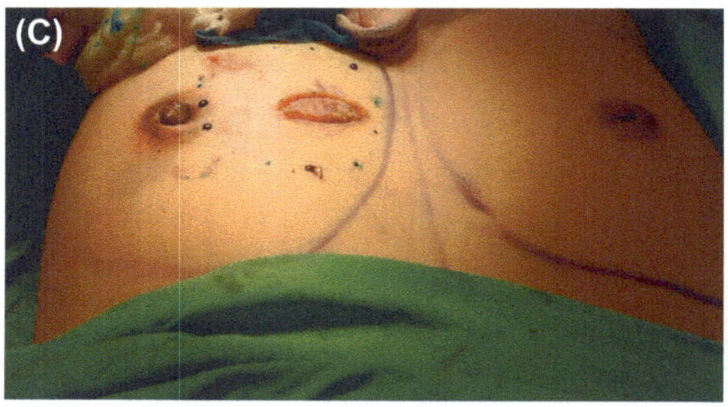

3.10C

On-table view showing markings of margins to be taken with blue dye. Skin overlying tumor was taken due to adherence of tumor to skin.

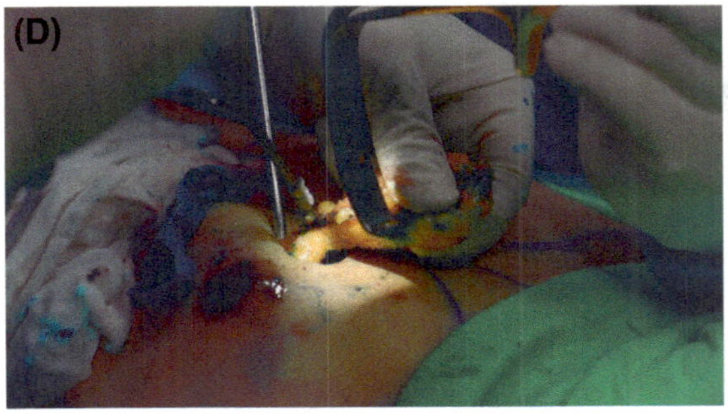

3.10D

Completion of wide excision with retraction technique.

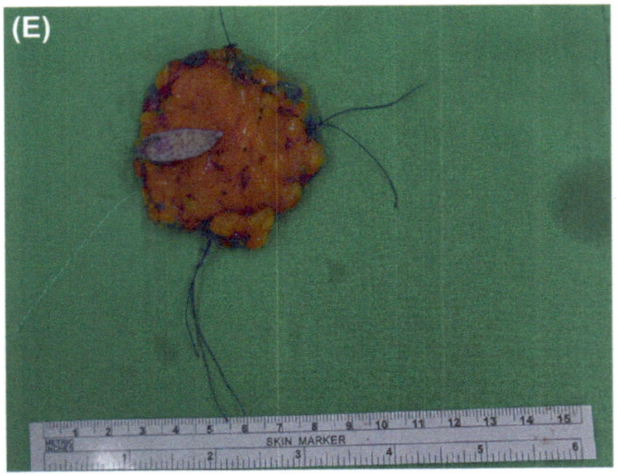

3.10E

Wide excision specimen as shown here with an ellipse of skin taken together.

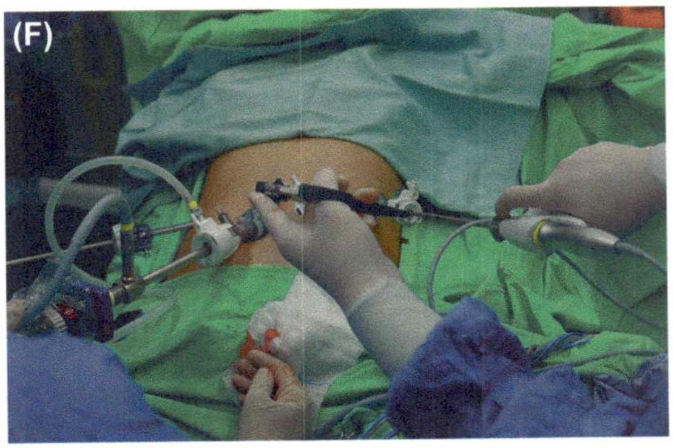

3.10F

Position of laparoscopic ports and instruments with surgeon standing on the patient's left with two working ports.

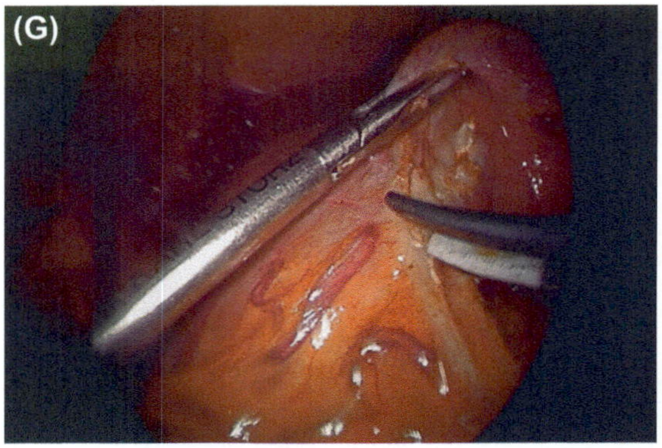

3.10G

Endoscopic view showing greater omentum taken close to the stomach with preservation of the right gastroepiploic vessels as the feeding vessels for the flap.

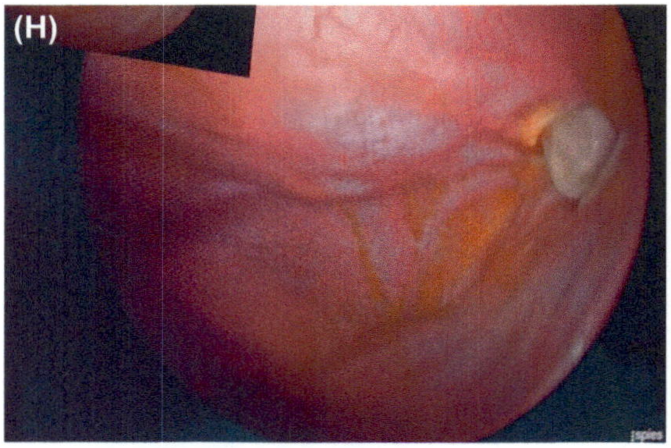

3.10H

Endoscopic view showing development of a window at the linea alba through which the pedicled flap was exteriorized.

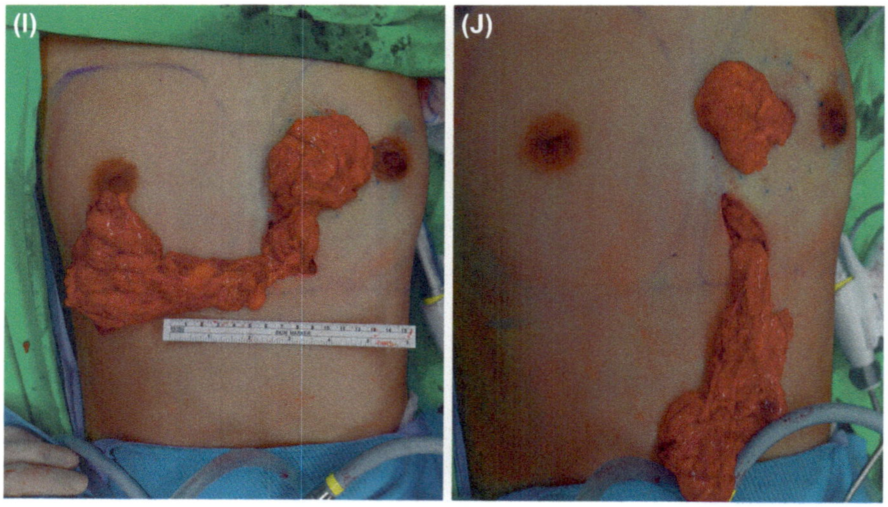

3.10I, J

Pedicled omental flap exteriorized and fashioned for reconstruction. The flap was further divided into two parts; one for partial breast reconstruction on the left and another for autologous breast augmentation on the right side.

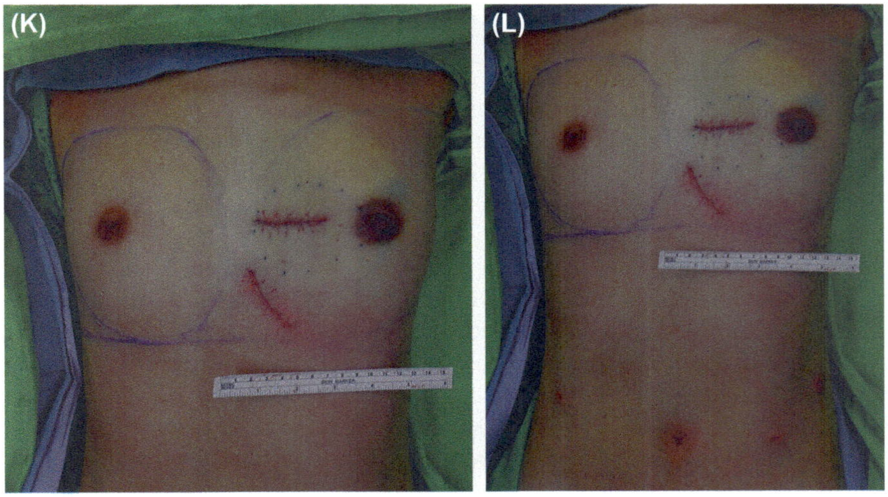

3.10K, L

Immediate post-operative views.

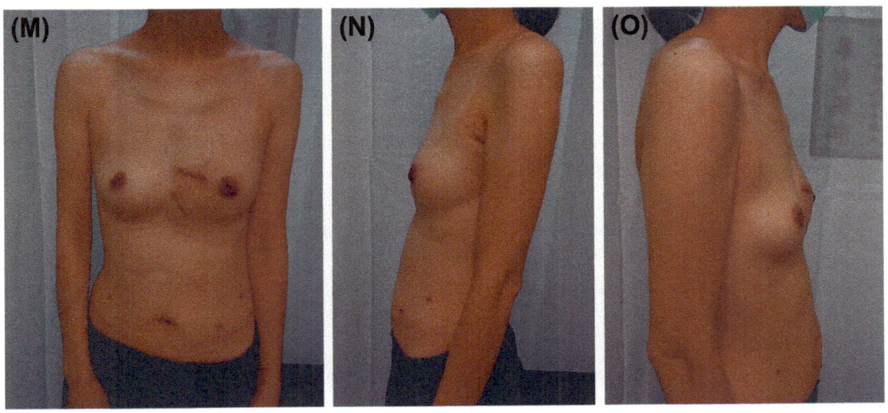

3.10M–O

Post-operative 2 weeks view in outpatient setting showing satisfactory volume replacement.

Discussion

Laparoscopic harvest of omentum as a partial breast reconstruction option has been gaining popularity over the past few years. The advantage of an omental flap lies in the fact that it is a vascular and robust flap with adequate volume up to moderate resection volume. In addition, studies have shown that omental flaps were shown to be resistant to post-radiotherapy flap volume loss or shrinkage (Khater, Fathi, & Ghazy, 2018). Considerations for patient selection include the absence of previous abdominal surgery to reduce the risk of complications from the donor site as well as informing the patient that the option will be abandoned should there be inadequate omentum for harvest and other alternative reconstruction options. Tumour suitable for an omental flap reconstruction would be tumour in the lower inner quadrant in view that a single medial inframammary skin crease incision would be adequate for both wide excision and flap harvest. However, tumours in other locations can also be offered volume replacement with a pedicled omental flap as long as the pedicle is long enough for the flap to be brought up into the cavity (Ni et al., 2018). For example, omentum flap has been shown to deliver excellent aesthetic outcomes in upper inner quadrant tumour, also known as 'the no man's land' of partial breast reconstruction (Zaha, H. et al., 2017). Care must be taken to ensure that the pedicle is not rotated during exteriorization. Omental flap has also been proven in terms of its oncological safety and technical feasibility from a recent review of the literature (Shash, Al-halabi, & Aldekhayel, 2018).

References

Khater, A., Fathi, A., & Ghazy, H. (2018). Omental flap in breast reconstruction. In *Issues in flap surgery*. https://doi.org/10.5772/intechopen.70115.

Ni, C., Zhu, Z., Xin, Y., Xie, Q., Yuan, H., Zhong, M., et al. (2018). Oncoplastic breast reconstruction with omental flap: A retrospective study and systematic review. *Journal of Cancer*. https://doi.org/10.7150/jca.25556.

Shash, H., Al-halabi, B., & Aldekhayel, S. (2018). Laparoscopic harvesting of omental flaps for breast reconstruction—a review of the literature and outcome analysis. *Plastic Surgery*. https://doi.org/10.1177/2292550317731762.

Zaha, H, et al. (2017). Oncoplastic surgery with omental flap reconstruction: a study of 200 cases. *Breast Cancer Research and Treatment*. https://doi.org/10.1007/s10549-017-4124-9.

CHAPTER

4

Endoscopic breast-conserving surgery with immediate local advancement/perforator flap reconstruction

Description of technique

Pre-operative marking and positioning

Pre-operative marking was done with the patient in standing and supine position. After induction of general anaesthesia, the patient was then placed in the supine position and ipsilateral arm raised above the ahead and secured to avoid affecting the operative procedure. Endoscopic video monitors (Olympus Optical Co., Tokyo, Japan) were set up on both sides of the patient's head to allow both the surgeon and the assistant to view the monitor. An oblique-ended rigid endoscope measuring 5 mm in diameter with a viewing angle of 30 degrees was used in all procedures. Pre-operative marking and design of the flap were performed, taking into consideration the location of intercostal artery perforator vessels using Doppler ultrasound. The lateral intercostal artery perforator (LiCAP) flap was used in the case discussion later.

Axillary staging procedure

In patients for whom sentinel lymph node biopsy (SLNB) is indicated, a small amount (2−3 mCi) of radioisotope Tc99m was injected intradermally at the site of the tumour before operation (either on the day or 1 day prior).

After induction of general anaesthesia, 3 mL of 1% methylene blue (Merck, Darmstadt, Germany) was injected into the breast parenchyma in equally divided aliquots at five positions surrounding the hemisphere of the tumour facing the ipsilateral axilla. The breast tissue from the tumour to the axilla was then gently massaged for 5−10 minutes. Within 20−30 minutes after injection of the blue dye, a handheld gamma probe (Navigator; USSC, Norwalk, CT) was used to identify the hot spots, and the location of the hottest nodes was then marked. An approximately 3-cm oblique axillary incision was then made close to the hottest nodes, and SLNB was then

Minimally Invasive (Endoscopic & Robotic) Breast Surgery. https://doi.org/10.1016/B978-0-323-73405-9.00004-2

performed. Fresh frozen section was performed as indicated. If SLN was positive for metastases, a complete axillary lymph node dissection up to level II was performed.

Development of flap and wide excision

After axillary staging procedure, incision was made along the superior aspect of the flap. A physiological saline solution containing lidocaine 0.05% and epinephrine 1: 1,000,000 was injected subcutaneously into the whole breast to minimize bleeding. An approximately 3–5-mm-thick skin flap was created via tunnelling method using an optical bladeless trocar Xcel (Johnson & Johnson, Tokyo, Japan) under endoscopic guidance. Subsequently, the septa between the skin flap and parenchyma was dissected and taken off under endoscopic guidance using endoscissors, bipolar scissors, or a harmonic scalpel.

An endoscopic Ultra Retractor (Johnson & Johnson KK or Karl Storz) vein harvester was used for the dissection pectoral muscle fascia off posterior portion of breast parenchyma. The penetrating vessels were coagulated and cut with bipolar scissors (PowerStar, Johnson & Johnson KK) or a harmonic scalpel to ensure adequate haemostasis and therefore better visual clarity. Counter traction was applied by retracting surrounding tissue with the Ultra Retractor under endoscopic guidance to create a sufficient working space, and a suction tube can be used to evacuate mist and smoke.

After development of adequate skin flap, wide excision was performed using bipolar or monopolar diathermy. To guide resection with adequate margins, the authors recommended the use of intra-operative ultrasound and marking of resection margin with blue dye injection. Specimen was retrieved thereafter and haemostasis secured.

Lateral intercostal artery perforator flap

After completion of wide excision, the next step involved raising the LiCAP flap and performing a level II oncoplastic reconstruction. The flap is raised based on the perforator vessels identified pre-op and marked with stitch intra-op. Care must be taken to ensure careful dissection of flap off fascia to avoid injuring the perforator vessels. After careful dissection and raising of flap, the flap was then de-epithelized and rotated around the pedicle into the resection cavity. Absorbable stitches were then placed to fix the flap. Drain was placed through the axillary incision, draining both axilla and resection cavity.

Case 11: endoscopic breast-conserving surgery with immediate local advancement/perforator flap reconstruction – lateral intercostal artery perforator flap

Patient/demographics

The patient is a 33-year-old lady with newly diagnosed clinical stage I left breast invasive ductal carcinoma, ER/PR+, CerbB2+. Pre-operative ultrasound revealed a 1.9cm tumour while pre-operative MRI Breast showed multiple satellite nodules around the primary lesion.

Her metastatic workup was negative.

Local advancement flap was offered to the patient as a partial reconstruction method, as the patient was particularly concerned with deformity after a wide excision but not keen for other reconstructive options.

Surgery and pathology report

This lady underwent an endoscopic breast-conserving surgery with sentinel lymph node biopsy and immediate lateral intercostal artery perforator (LiCAP) flap reconstruction. The frozen section for sentinel lymph node biopsy was negative.

Her final histopathology was a stage 1 disease, T1cN0M0.

Post-operative outcomes

The patient recovered well with no complications encountered. She also received adjuvant radiotherapy and endocrine therapy for 5 years.

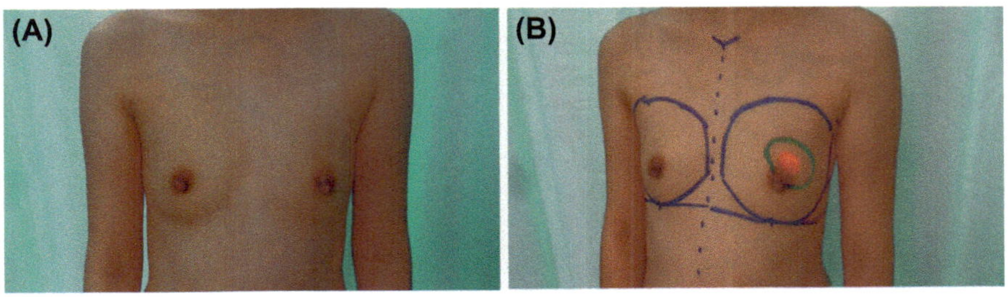

4.11A, B

Pre-operative front views showing pre-operative markings and location of tumor.

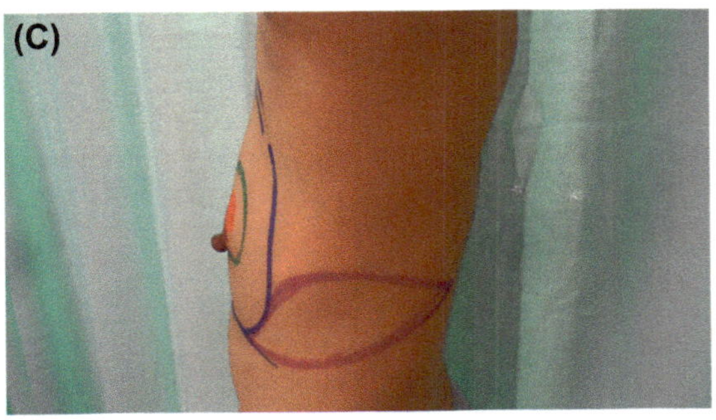

4.11C

Markings of LiCAP flap pre-operatively.

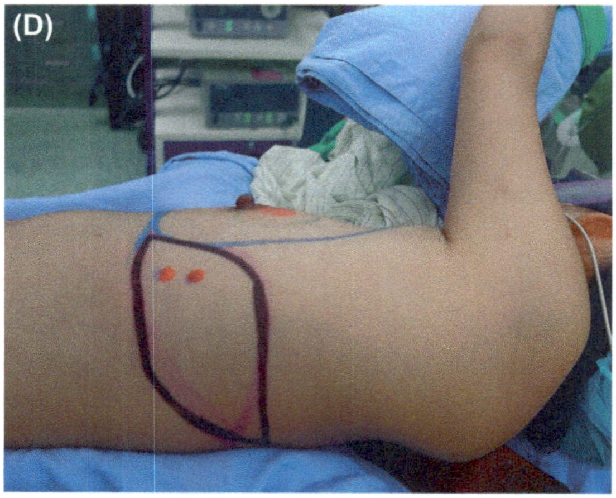

4.11D

On-table view showing position of patient with ipsilateral upper limb held above head on an armrest.

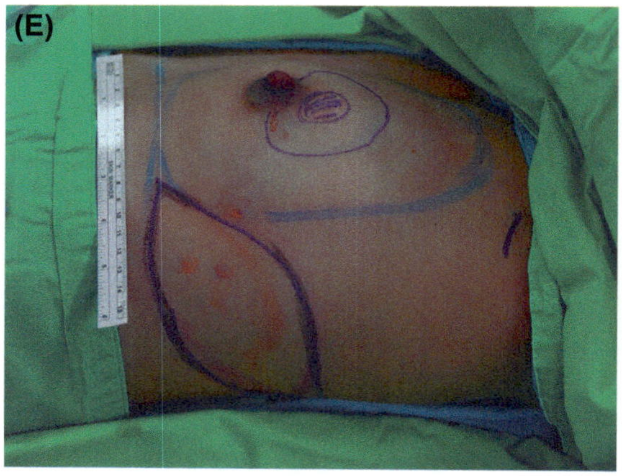

4.11E

Incisions planned as shown above (axillary skin crease incision for sentinel lymph node biopsy and incision over superior part of LiCAP flap for wide excision).

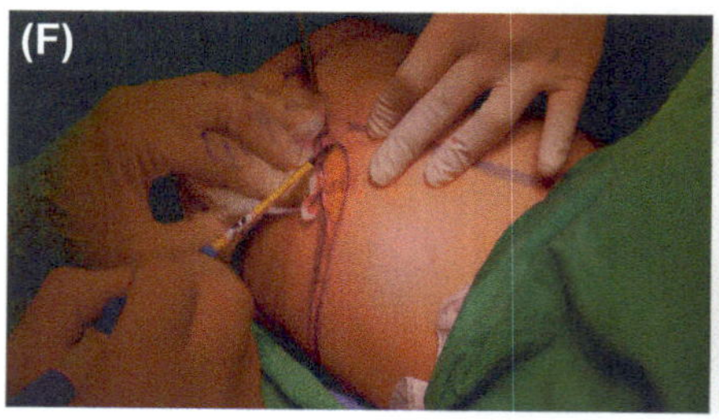

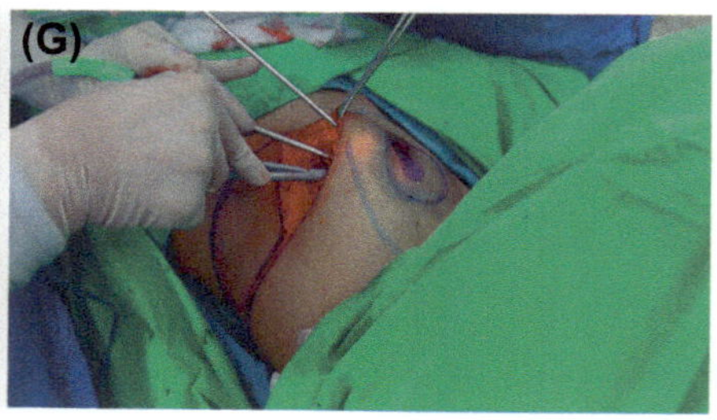

4.11F, G

After sentinel lymph node biopsy, wide excision performed via incision over superior part of LiCAP flap.

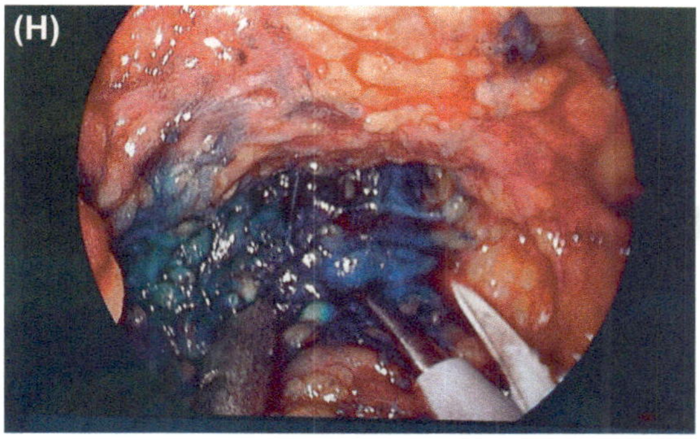

4.11H

Endoscopic view showing dissection of skin flap off the parenchyma.

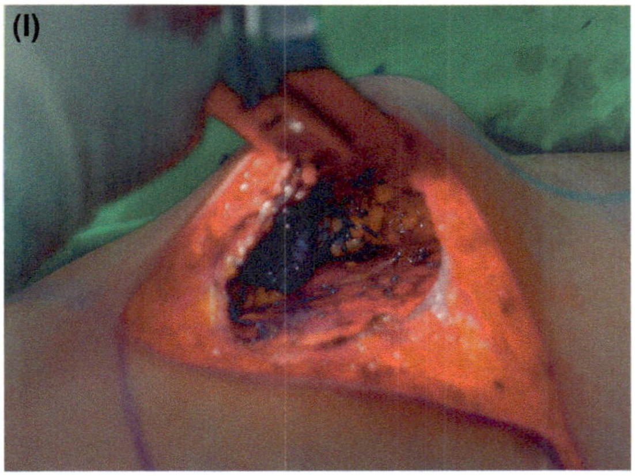

4.11I

Resection cavity seen under direct vision after wide excision specimen retrieved.

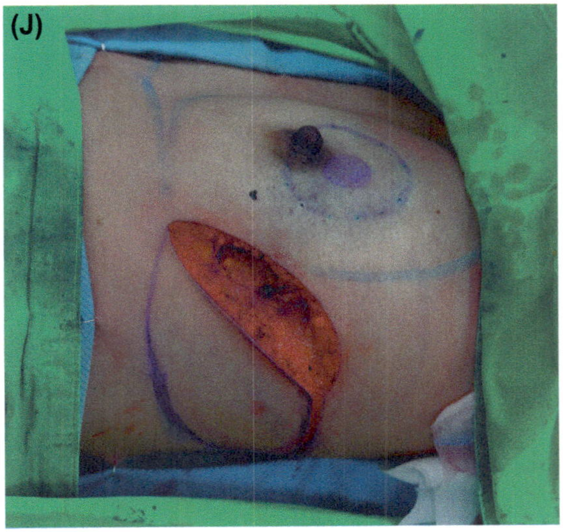

4.11J

On-table view after wide excision.

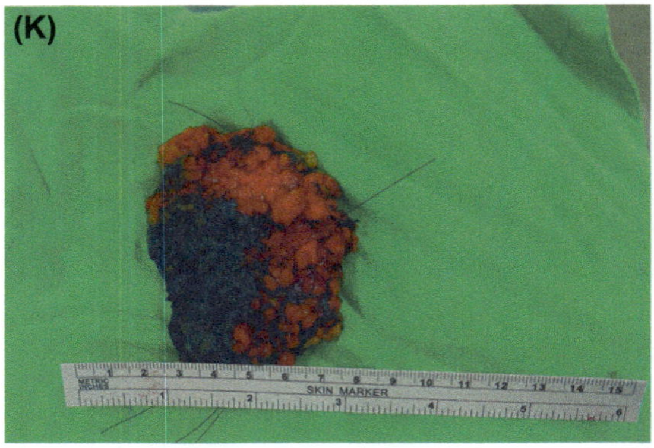

4.11K

Wide excision specimen retrieved as a whole and oriented.

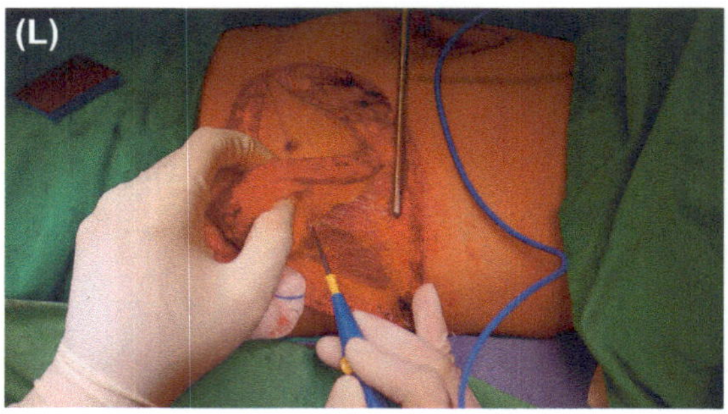

4.11L

LiCAP flap raised all the way to muscle fascia along perforator vessels marked pre-operatively.

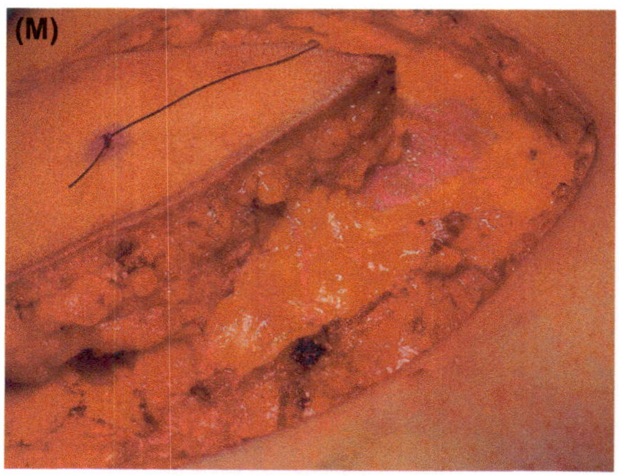

4.11M

A stitch was placed to mark the site of perforator vessels marked pre-operatively with Doppler ultrasound.

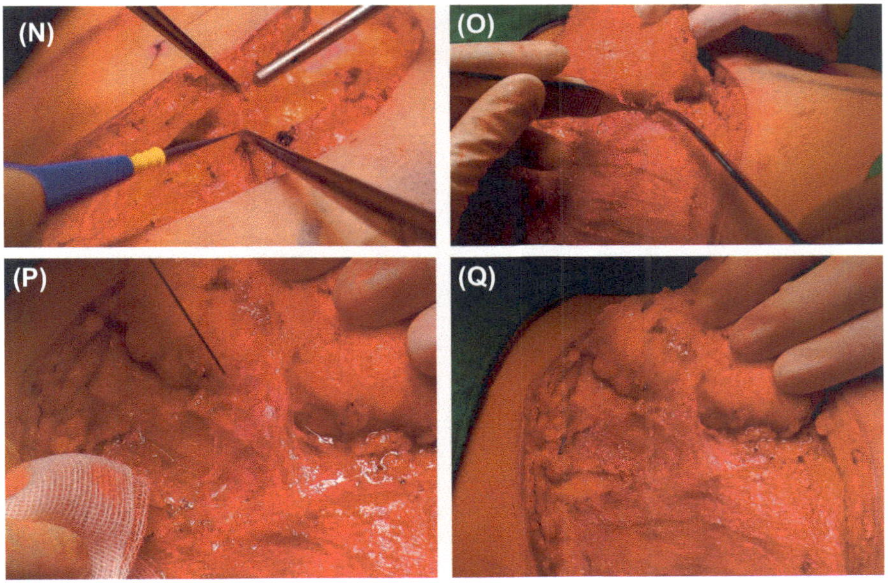

4.11N–Q

Perforator vessels meticulously identified, dissected, and isolated free.

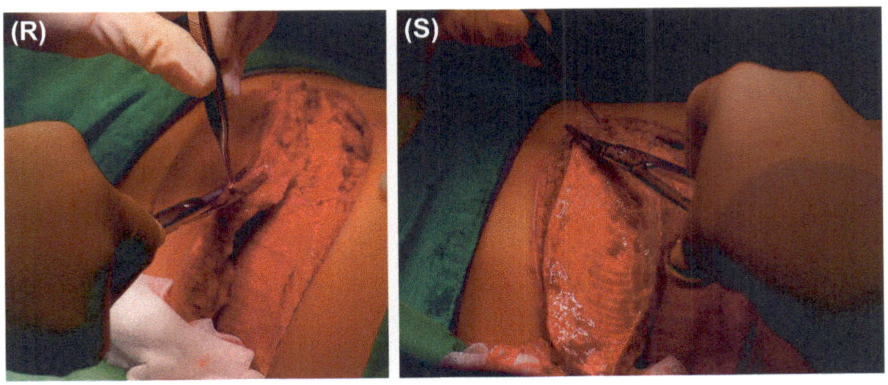

4.11R, S

LiCAP flap de-epitheliazed before reconstruction.

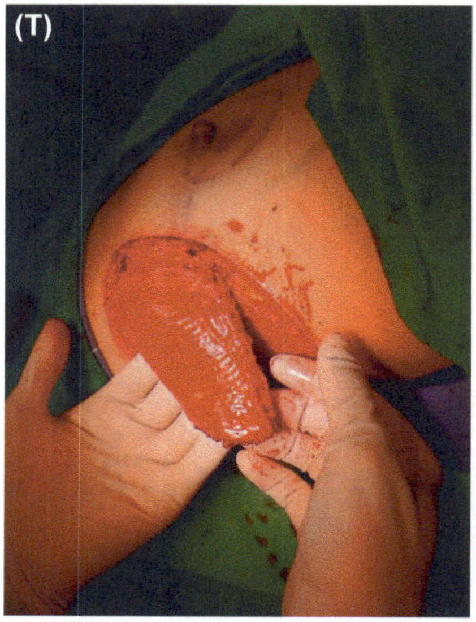

4.11T

LiCAP flap complete raised and epitheliazed.

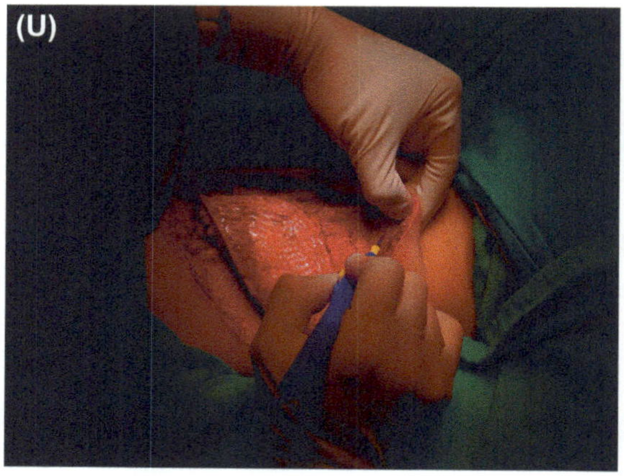

4.11U

Breast tissue mobilized before level II oncoplastic procedure performed with LiCAP flap.

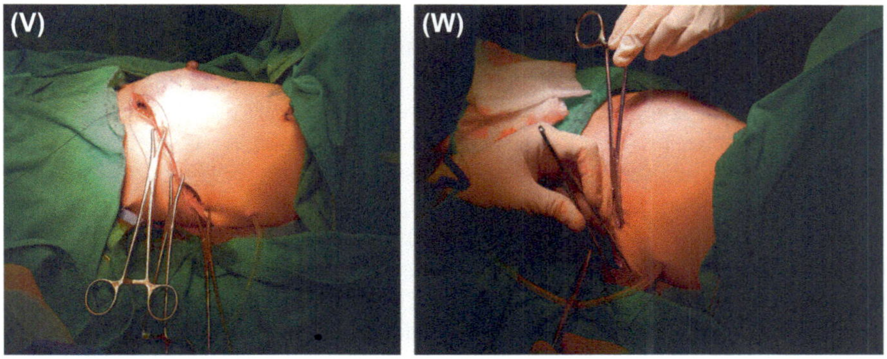

4.11V, W

Incisions approximated to ensure tension free closure in layers.

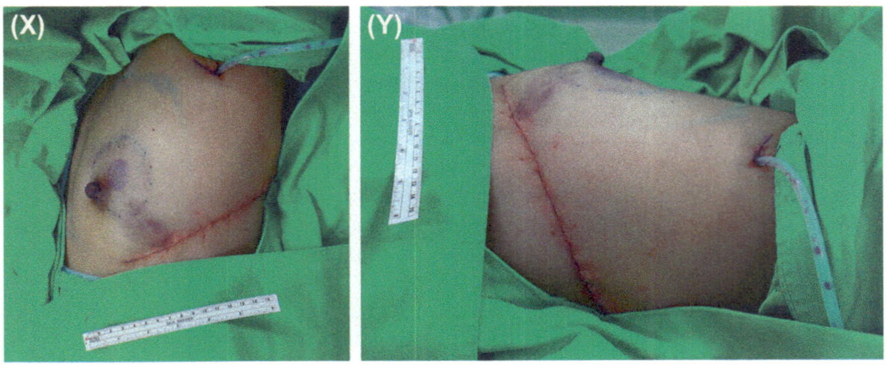

4.11X, Y

Immediate on-table post-operative views.

Discussion

LiCAP flap is a great volume replacement technique for a partial reconstruction after a breast-conserving surgery. As with most level II oncoplastic procedures, this technique is suitable for a moderate resection volume post-wide excision and is commonly performed for tumours located in the outer portion of the breast. Selection criteria for this technique other than tumour location would include important patient characteristics (no major co-morbidities, no known cardiovascular or peripheral vascular disease, non-smoker) to ensure its success (Macmillan & McCulley, 2016). Pre-operative identification of perforator vessels is essential and holds the key to success of this operation. The authors suggest pre-operative and intra-operative bedside Doppler ultrasound for identification of perforator vessels. Placing a stitch over marked Doppler identification point will help in subsequent detection intra-op. A recent systematic review suggested the use of colour Doppler ultrasound for better pre-operative planning with wider margins of safety and better reproducibility (Sørensen, Ibrahim, Gunnarsson, Akram, & Thomsen, 2018). A LiCAP flap does not require post-operative flap monitoring, but intra-operative identification of a healthy flap includes bleeding from flap edges upon re-fashioning and de-epithelization. The downside of this technique may arise from the long incision from the donor site; hence, the incision should be planned along the line where it will be within the undergarment line or hidden under the arm (Kim et al., 2018).

References

Kim, J. B., Kim, D. K., Lee, J. W., Choi, K. Y., Chung, H. Y., Cho, B. C., et al. (2018). The usefulness of pedicled perforator flap in partial breast reconstruction after breast conserving surgery in Korean women. *Archives of Plastic Surgery*. https://doi.org/10.5999/aps.2017.01200.

Macmillan, R. D., & McCulley, S. J. (2016). Oncoplastic breast surgery: What, when and for whom? *Current Breast Cancer Reports*. https://doi.org/10.1007/s12609-016-0212-9.

Sørensen, J. A., Ibrahim, R. M., Gunnarsson, G. L., Akram, J., & Thomsen, J. B. (2018). Color Doppler ultrasonography targeted reconstruction using pedicled perforator flaps—a systematic review and meta-analysis. *European Journal of Plastic Surgery*. https://doi.org/10.1007/s00238-018-1435-y.

SECTION

3

Endoscopic mastectomy with immediate reconstruction

CHAPTER

Endoscopic mastectomy with immediate implant reconstruction

5

Description of technique

Pre-operative marking and positioning

Pre-operative marking was done with the patient in standing and supine position. After induction of general anaesthesia, the patient was then placed in the supine position and ipsilateral arm abducted to 90 degrees to avoid affecting the operative procedure. Endoscopic video monitors (Olympus Optical Co., Tokyo, Japan) were set up on both sides of the patient's head to allow both the surgeon and the assistant to view the monitor. An oblique-ended rigid endoscope measuring 5 mm in diameter with a viewing angle of 30 degrees was used in all procedures.

Axillary staging procedure

In patients for whom sentinel lymph node biopsy (SLNB) is indicated, a small amount (2−3 mCi) of radioisotope Tc99m was injected intradermally at the site of the tumour before operation (either on the day or 1 day prior).

After induction of general anaesthesia, 3 mL of 1% methylene blue (Merck, Darmstadt, Germany) was injected into the breast parenchyma in equally divided aliquots at five positions surrounding the hemisphere of the tumour facing the ipsilateral axilla. The breast tissue from the tumour to the axilla was then gently massaged for 5−10 minutes. Within 20−30 minutes after injection of the blue dye, a handheld gamma probe (Navigator; USSC, Norwalk, CT) was used to identify the hot spots, and the location of the hottest nodes was then marked. An approximately 3-cm oblique axillary incision was then made close to the hottest nodes, and SLNB was then performed. Fresh frozen section was performed as indicated. If SLN was positive for metastases, a complete axillary lymph node dissection up to level II was performed.

Dissection of breast parenchyma off pectoralis major fascia

After completion of axillary staging procedure, dissection was carried out to the lateral border of the pectoralis major muscle. The margin between pectoralis muscle and breast parenchyma was clearly identified. An endoscopic Ultra Retractor

Minimally Invasive (Endoscopic & Robotic) Breast Surgery. https://doi.org/10.1016/B978-0-323-73405-9.00005-4

(Johnson & Johnson KK or Karl Storz) vein harvester was used for the dissection pectoral muscle fascia off posterior portion of breast parenchyma. The penetrating vessels were coagulated and cut with bipolar scissors (PowerStar, Johnson & Johnson KK) or a harmonic scalpel to ensure adequate haemostasis and therefore better visual clarity. Counter traction was applied by retracting surrounding tissue with the Ultra Retractor under endoscopic guidance to create a sufficient working space, and a suction tube can be used to evacuate mist and smoke.

Placement of single port, tunnelling and development of skin flap (in cases of endoscopic mastectomy with insufflation technique)

To create a working space for the placement of the single port (Glove Port; Nelis Corporation, Gyeonggi-do, Korea), a 3–4 cm subcutaneous flap was dissected with electrocautery under direct vision. Once adequate dissection was achieved, the single port was then inserted through the axilla incision, and carbon dioxide (CO_2) insufflation with air pressure kept at 8 mmHg was used to create space for mastectomy. Dissection was then continued from the superficial skin flaps by dissecting the septa between the skin flap and parenchyma created by the tunnelling technique with monopolar scissors. A sub-areolar biopsy and fresh frozen section analysis can be performed in a nipple-sparing mastectomy. If cancer cell invasion was found in the sub-areolar area, the entire nipple-areolar complex (NAC) was removed and conversion to a skin-sparing mastectomy was then performed. After completion of the superficial skin flap dissection, dissection of the peripheral portion of the breast parenchyma was carried out subsequently. After completion of dissection, the entire breast specimen was removed through the axillary wound.

Tunnelling and development of skin flap (in cases of endoscopic mastectomy with retraction technique)

After completion of the axillary staging procedure, a semi-circular peri-areolar skin incision or a single axillary incision was made (depending on surgeon's preference) as previously described. A physiological saline solution containing lidocaine 0.05% and epinephrine 1:1,000,000 was injected subcutaneously into the whole breast to minimize bleeding. An approximately 3–5-mm-thick skin flap was created via tunnelling method using an optical bladeless trocar Xcel (Johnson & Johnson, Tokyo, Japan) under endoscopic guidance. Subsequently, the septa between the skin flap and parenchyma was dissected and taken off under endoscopic guidance using endoscissors, bipolar scissors, or a harmonic scalpel.

Mastectomy

Following adequate skin flap development, a sub-areolar biopsy and fresh frozen section analysis can be performed in a nipple-sparing mastectomy. If cancer cell invasion was found in the sub-areolar area, the entire NAC was removed and conversion to a skin-sparing mastectomy was then performed. After completion of skin flap development as well as detaching the breast off the pectoralis major fascia, the entire breast specimen can be removed via the axillary or peri-areolar incisions.

Immediate implant reconstruction

Following removal of the specimen and adequate haemostasis, copious irrigation of the mastectomy pocket was performed. Subsequently, the lateral border of the pectoralis major muscle was elevated to allow for submuscular pocket dissection. Dissection was performed medially towards the sternal border, taking care not to injure the perforator vessels. Inferiorly, the dissection was carried out beyond the inframammary fold (IMF) over the lateral aspect, below which the muscle was released to continue the dissection to the subcutaneous plane thus allowing for a more natural placement of the implant. In the lateral border, the superficial fascia of the serratus anterior muscle was dissected posteriorly in a limited fashion so that it was just enough to accommodate the lateral border of the implant. An implant (Mentor Worldwide LLC, Santa Barbara, CA) was then placed followed by drains placement in both submuscular and subcutaneous planes. Care was taken when tagging the free muscle edges laterally.

Case 12: Endoscopic nipple-sparing mastectomy with immediate implant reconstruction – single incision, retraction technique

Patient/demographics

This is a case of a 53-year-old lady with a 2.5 cm tumor in her left breast. Core biopsy pre-operatively revealed a ductal carcinoma in situ. The patient opted for a mastectomy and was keen for upfront reconstruction. She was not keen for autologous tissue but chose to have an implant reconstruction instead.

Her metastatic workup was negative.

Surgery and pathology report

The patient underwent an endoscopic nipple-sparing mastectomy with sentinel lymph node biopsy and immediate implant reconstruction. Intra-operative frozen section for sentinel lymph node and sub-nipple biopsy were both negative for metastases.

Her final histology showed residual DCIS (TisN0M0), and she did not receive any adjuvant therapy thereafter.

Post-operative outcomes

Her hospitalization was uneventful, and there were no immediate complications encountered. The patient was satisfied with her post-operative cosmesis when she was reviewed in outpatient clinic.

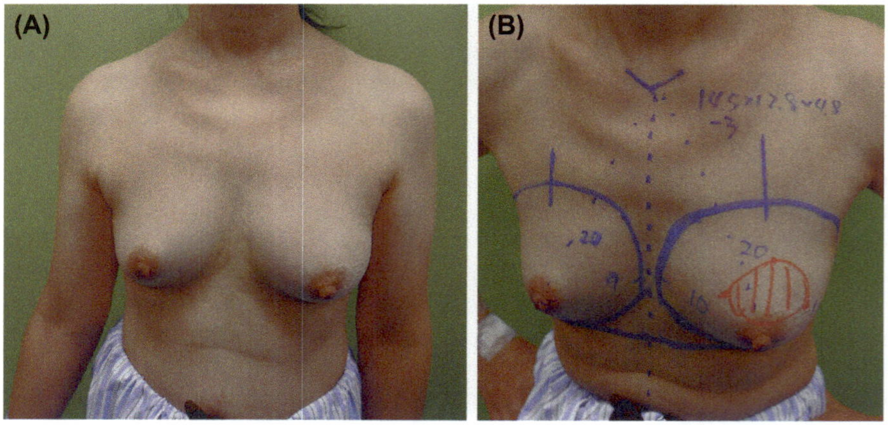

5.12A, B

Pre-operative front views showing pre-operative markings and location of tumor

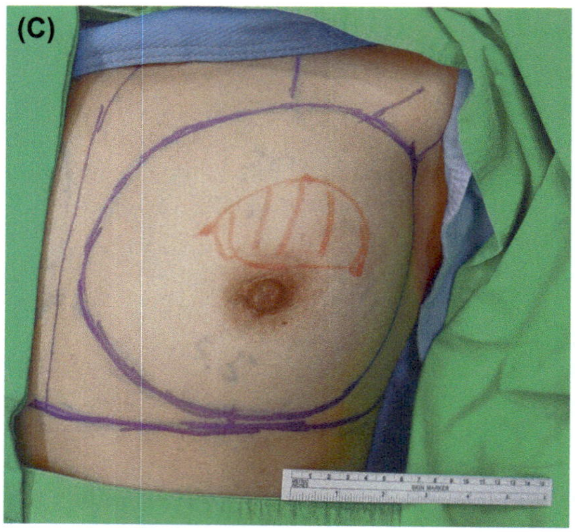

5.12C

On-table markings showing location of tumor and planned axillary incision

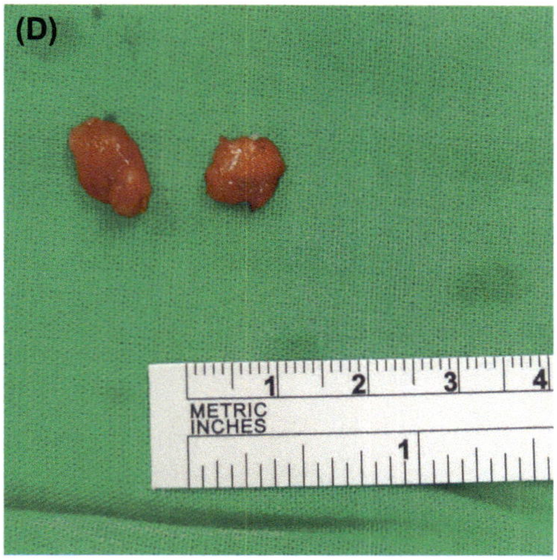

5.12D

Sentinel lymph nodes identified via dual modality

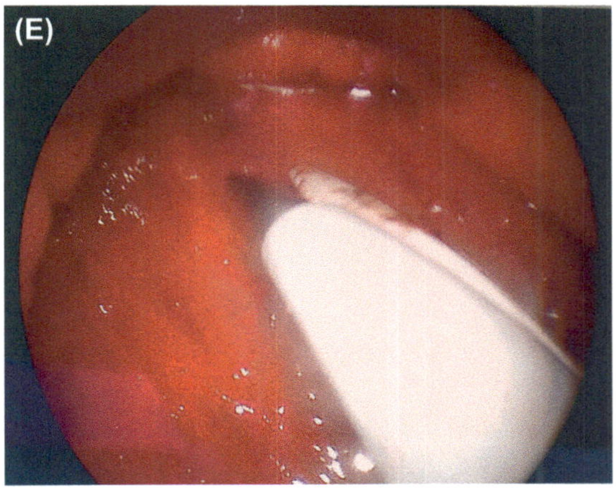

5.12E

Endoscopic Ultra Retractor (Johnson & Johnson KK or Karl Storz) vein harvester used for the dissection of pectoral muscle fascia off posterior portion of breast parenchyma

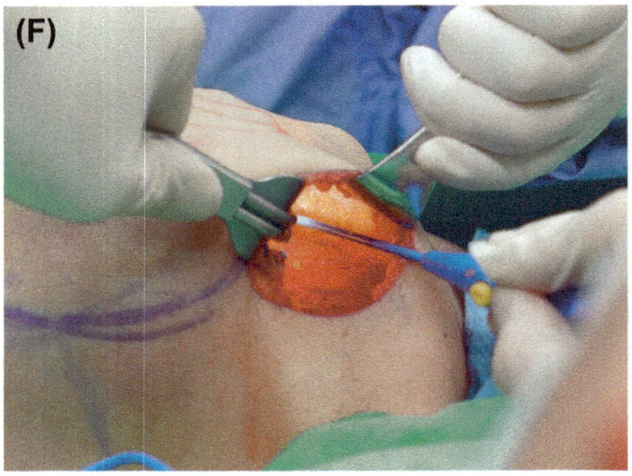

5.12F

Development of skin flap with the help of retractor and light source

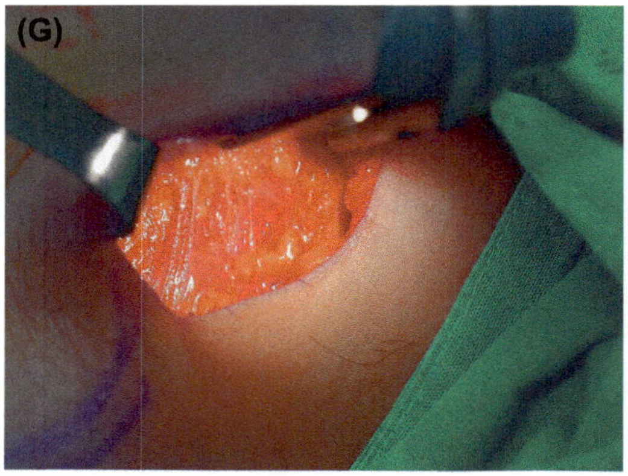

5.12G

Septa between skin flap and breast parenchyma visualized clearly

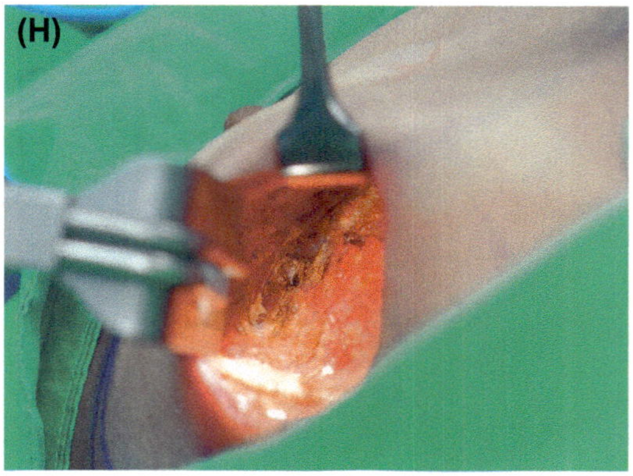

5.12H

Resection cavity seen under direct vision after mastectomy

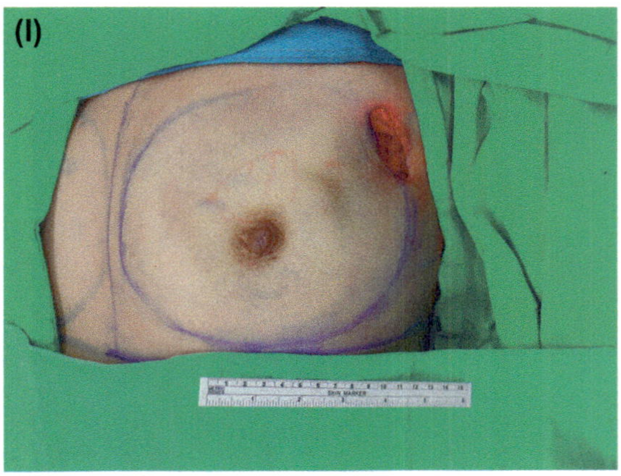

5.12I

On-table view after mastectomy

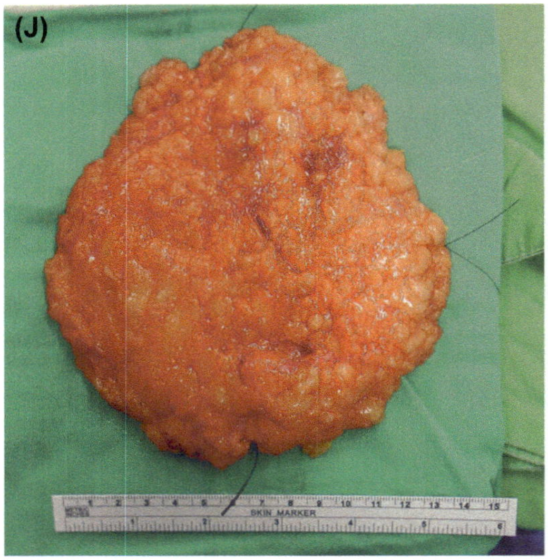

5.12J

Mastectomy specimen oriented with silk sutures

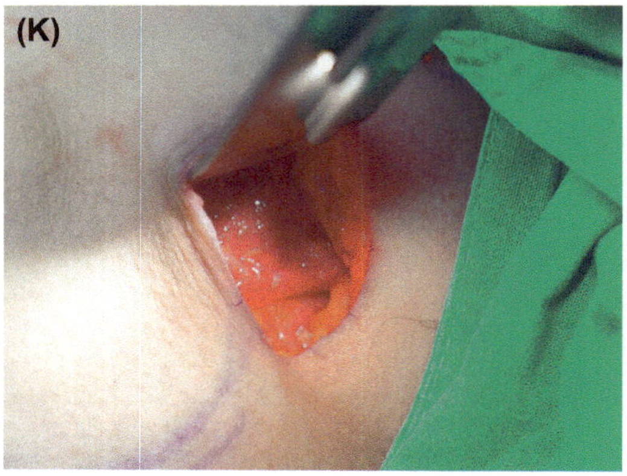

5.12K

Subpectoral pocket dissection started from the border of the pectoralis major muscle

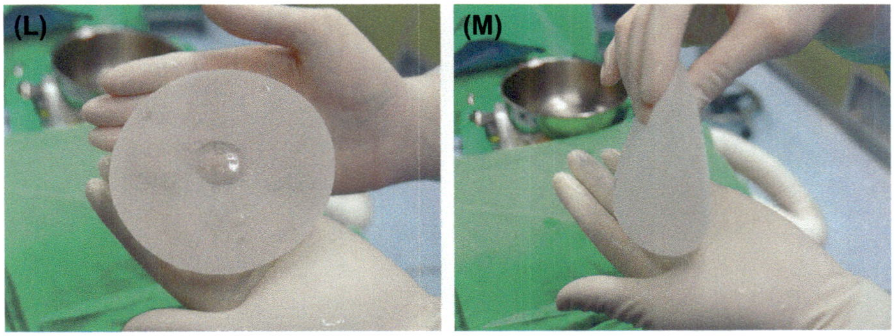

5.12L, M

Implant of a suitable size chosen for immediate reconstruction

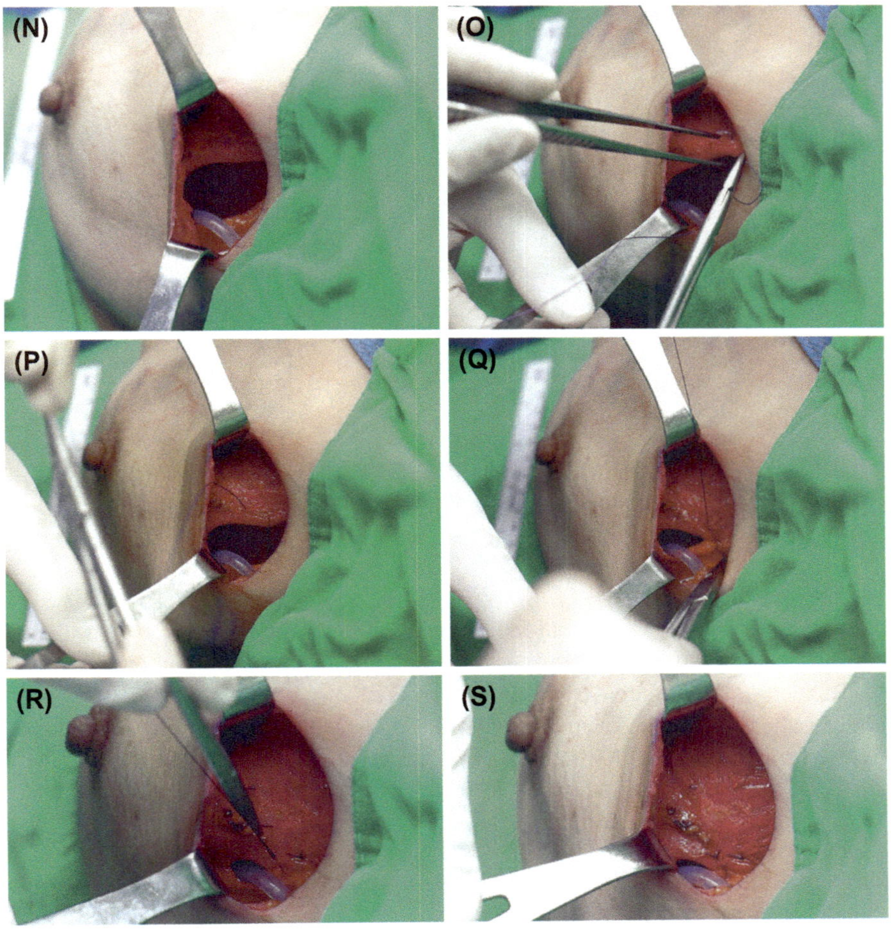

5.12N–S

Placement of implant and closure of the lateral border with approximation of pectoralis major muscle to serratus anterior with continuous absorbable sutures and drain placement thereafter

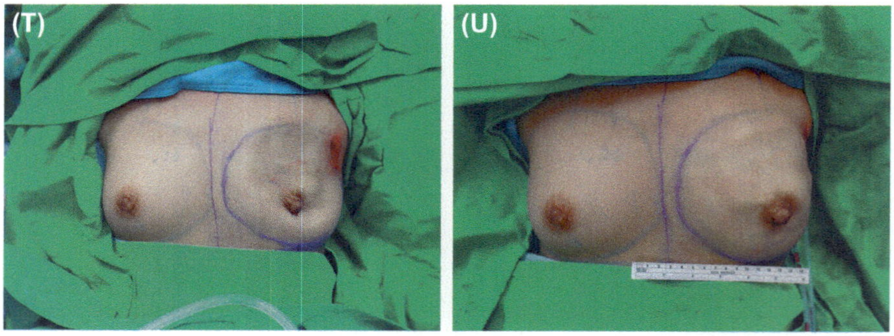

5.12T, U

On-table views before (t) and after (u) implant placement

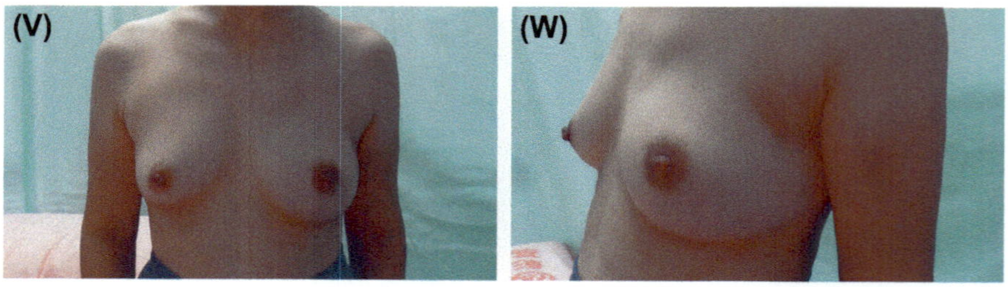

5.12V, W

1-year post-operative views showing excellent cosmesis and projection

Case 13: Endoscopic nipple-sparing mastectomy with immediate implant reconstruction – bilateral, retraction technique

Patient/demographics

The case described a 36-year-old lady diagnosed with clinical stage 0 right breast cancer with a pre-operative core biopsy report of a ductal carcinoma in situ.

Her metastatic workup did not reveal any distant metastases.

The patient was keen for right nipple-sparing mastectomy and contralateral prophylactic mastectomy with immediate implant reconstruction.

Surgery and pathology report

The patient underwent bilateral nipple-sparing mastectomy, right sentinel lymph node biopsy with bilateral immediate implant reconstruction. Right sentinel lymph node biopsy and bilateral sub-nipple biopsies for the frozen section were negative.

Final histology returned as right breast DCIS (TisN0M0), whereas the left breast only showed fibrocystic change and usual ductal hyperplasia. She did not receive further adjuvant therapy.

Post-operative outcomes

The patient was satisfied with her cosmesis, and there were no immediate complications encountered post-operatively.

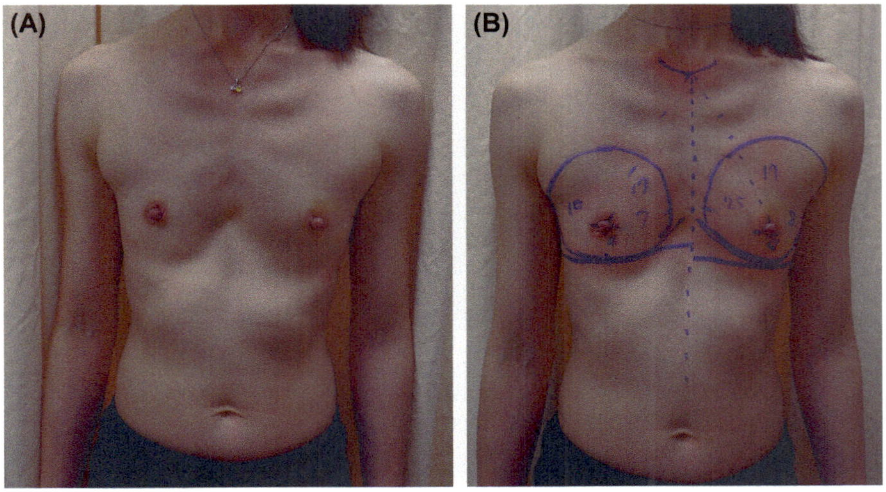

5.13A, B

Pre-operative front views showing pre-operative markings and location of tumor

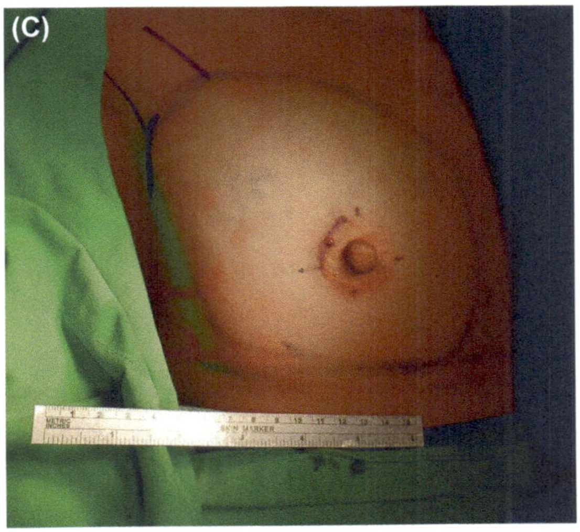

5.13C

On-table markings showing planned incisions over the right breast (dual incision - periareolar and axilla)

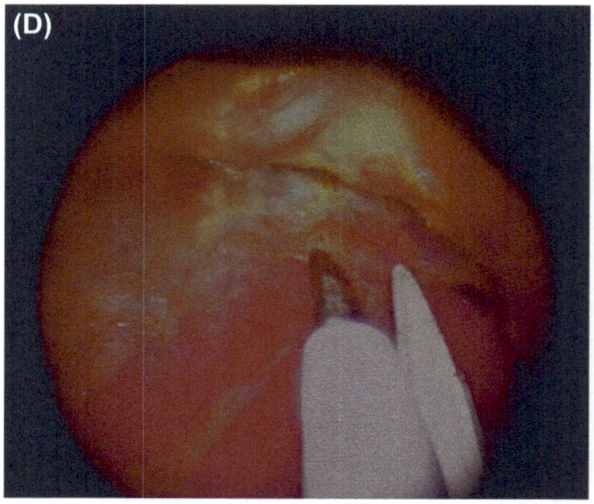

5.13D

Endoscopic Ultra Retractor (Johnson & Johnson KK or Karl Storz) vein harvester used for the dissection of pectoral muscle fascia off posterior portion of breast parenchyma

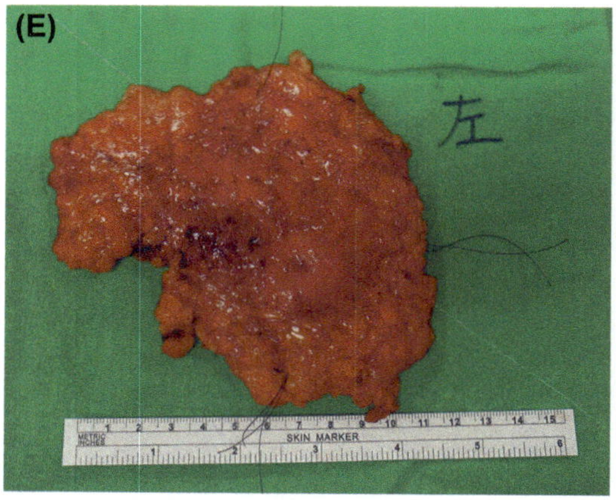

5.13E

Right mastectomy specimen

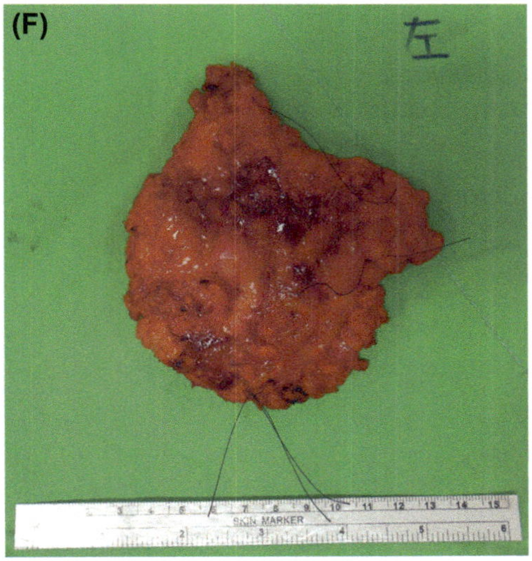

5.13F

Left mastectomy specimen

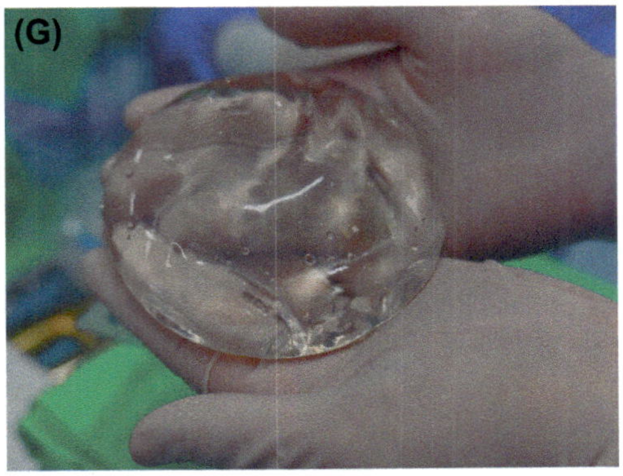

5.13G

Smooth implant for immediate reconstruction

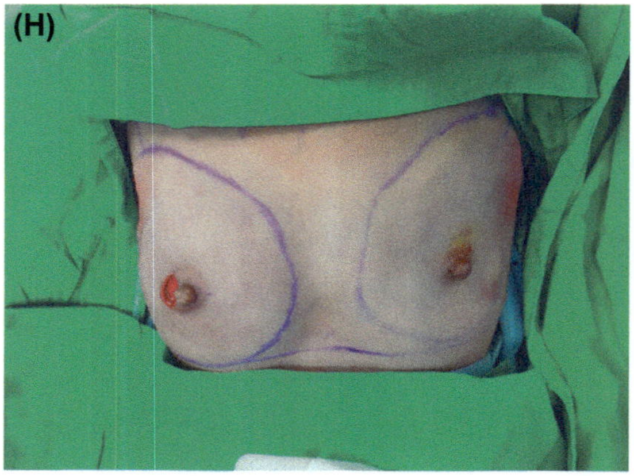

5.13H

Immediate on-table view before reconstruction

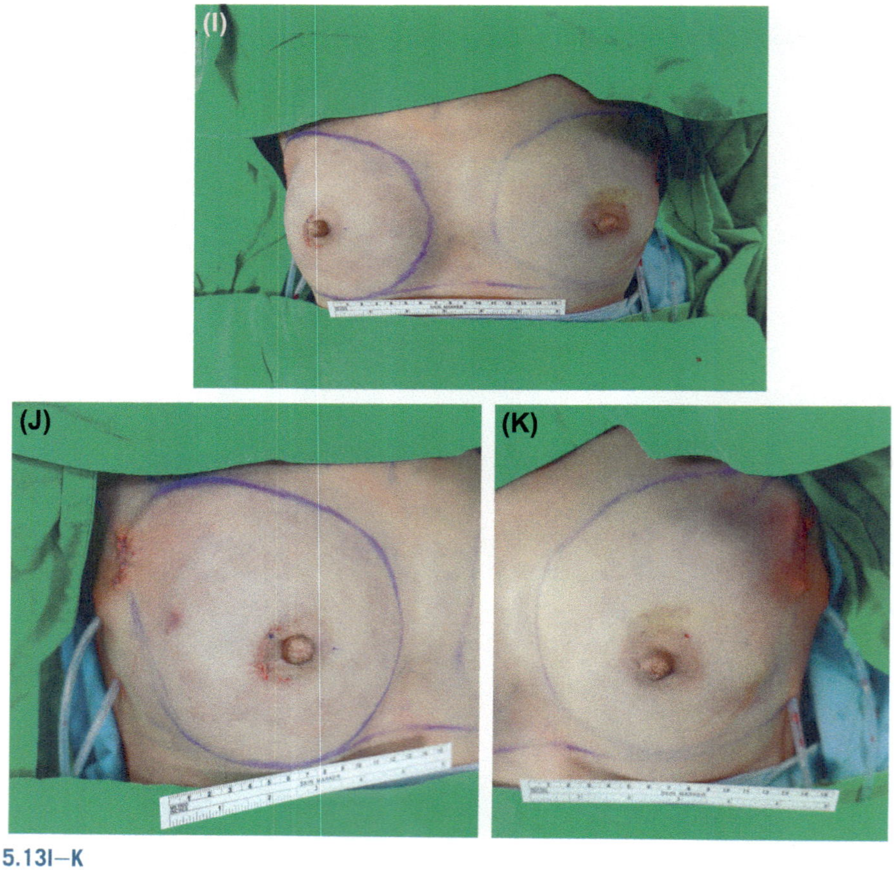

5.13I–K

On-table view after bilateral implant reconstruction with closed up views showing bilateral axillary and right peri-areolar incisions

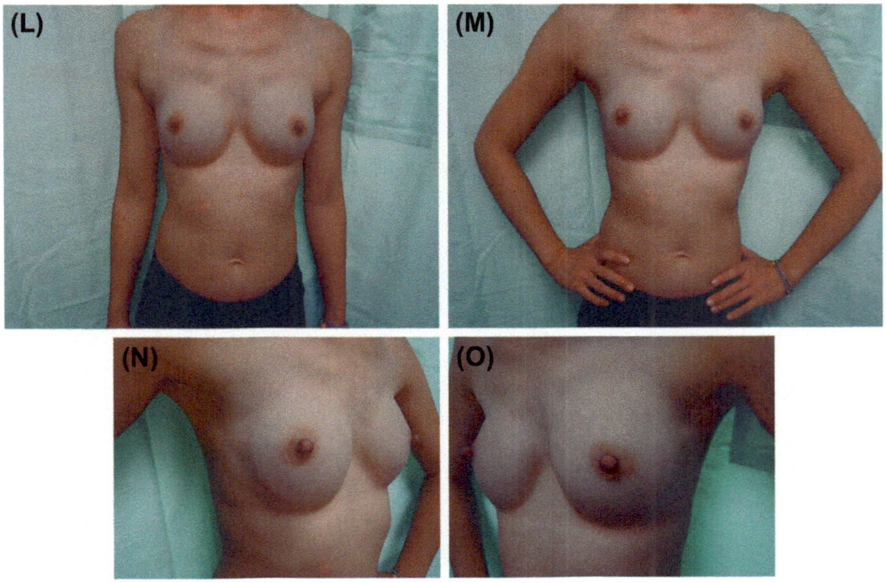

5.13L–O

Post-operative views 1 year after operation showing well-healed and well-hidden scars leading to excellent cosmesis

Case 14: Endoscopic nipple-sparing mastectomy with immediate implant reconstruction – bilateral, retraction technique

Patient/demographics

The case described a 48-year-old lady diagnosed with bilateral clinical stage I and 0 breast cancer for right side and left side, respectively. Pre-operative core biopsy revealed a right breast invasive lobular carcinoma and a left breast ductal carcinoma in situ.

Her metastatic workup did not reveal any distant metastases.

The patient was keen for bilateral nipple sparing mastectomy with immediate implant reconstruction at the same sitting.

Surgery and pathology report

The patient underwent bilateral nipple sparing mastectomy and sentinel lymph node biopsy with bilateral immediate implant reconstruction. Bilateral sentinel lymph node biopsy and sub-nipple biopsies for the frozen section were negative.

Final histology returned as right breast invasive lobular carcinoma with lobular carcinoma in situ (T1cN0M0), whereas the left breast was upstaged to invasive ductal carcinoma with ductal carcinoma in situ (T1aN0M0). The patient received endocrine therapy for 5 years.

Post-operative outcomes

This lady was discharged 2 days after operation, and no immediate complications were encountered.

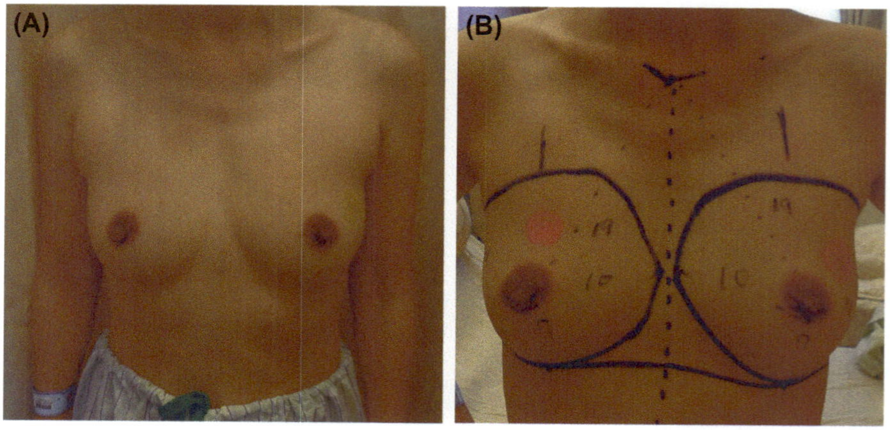

5.14A, B

Pre-operative front views showing pre-operative markings and location of tumor

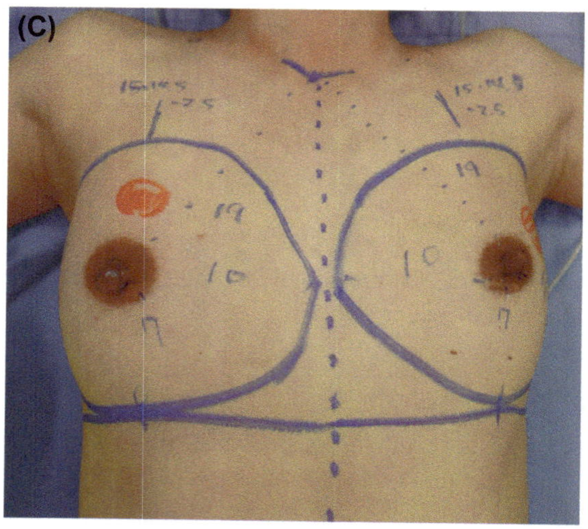

5.14C

On-table markings showing planned incisions over bilateral breast (bilateral single axillary incision)

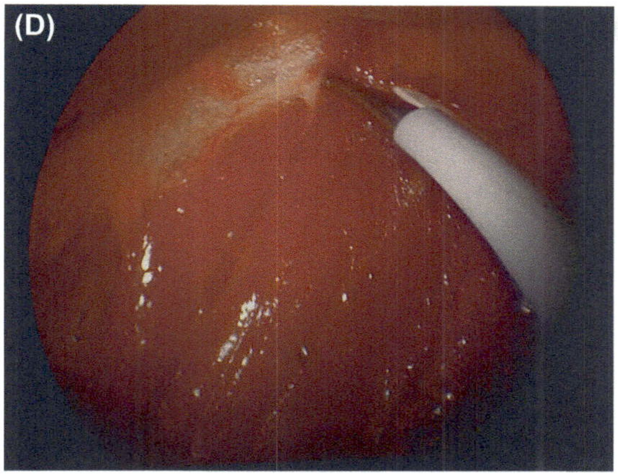

5.14D

Endoscopic Ultra Retractor (Johnson & Johnson KK or Karl Storz) vein harvester used for the dissection of pectoral muscle fascia off posterior portion of breast parenchyma

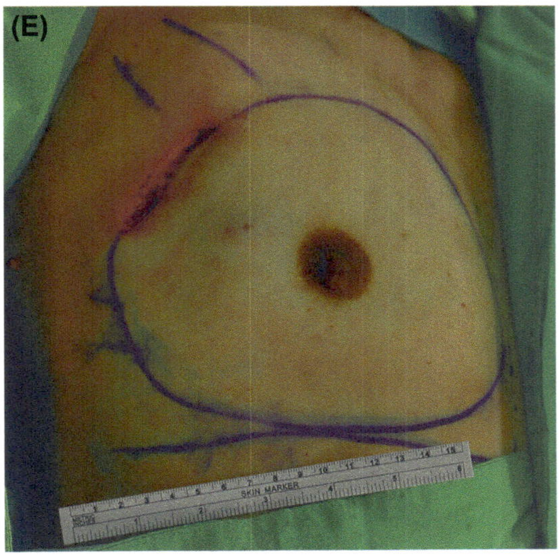

5.14E

Immediate view after right mastectomy

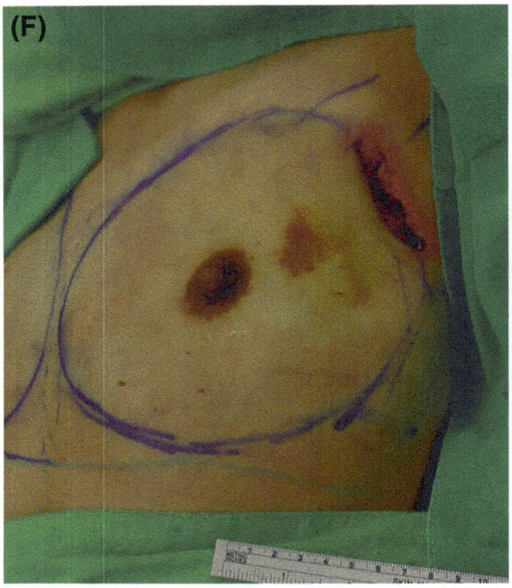

5.14F

Immediate view after left mastectomy

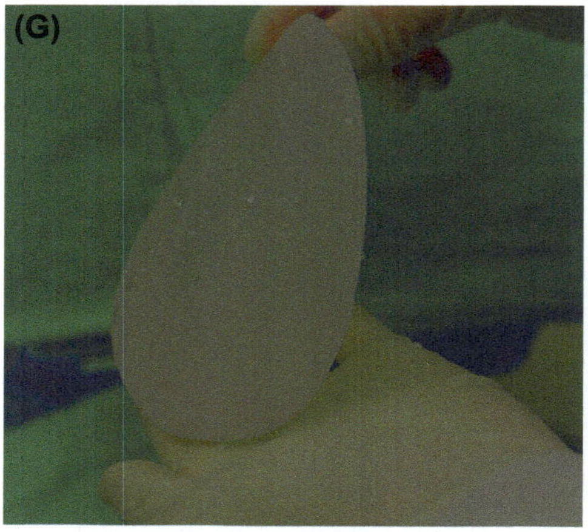

5.14G

Anatomical implant used for bilateral reconstruction

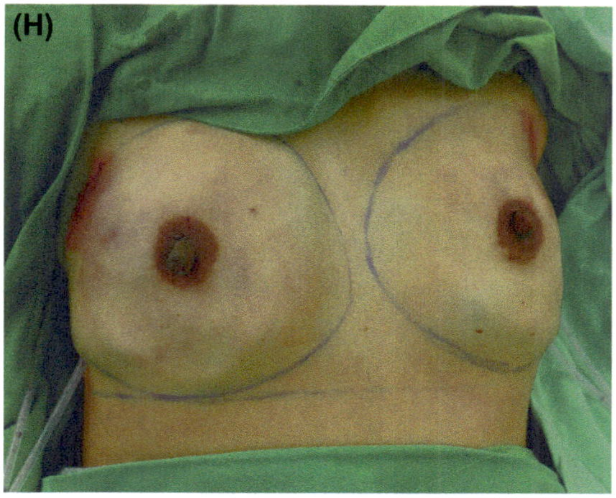

5.14H

Immediate on-table view before reconstruction

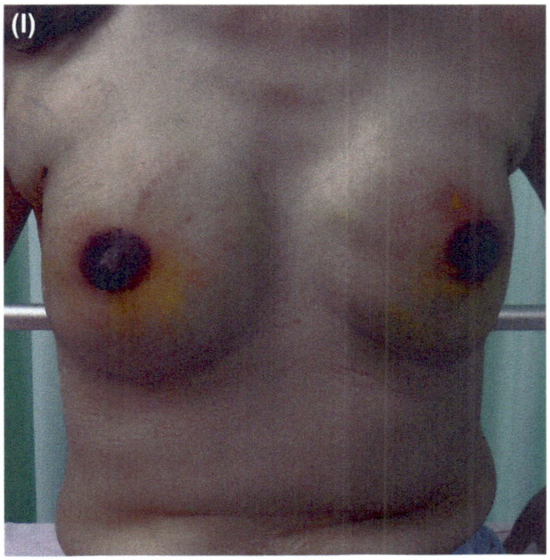

5.14I

2 weeks post-operative front view showing mild bruising. Note that both axillary incisions were well hidden beneath axillary breast

Case 15: Three-dimensional (3D) endoscopic nipple-sparing mastectomy with immediate implant reconstruction – single incision, insufflation technique

Patient/demographics

This is a case of a 42-year-old lady with a 3-cm tumor in her left breast. Core biopsy pre-operatively revealed an invasive ductal carcinoma and ductal carcinoma in situ. The patient opted for a mastectomy and was keen for upfront implant reconstruction.

Her metastatic workup was negative.

Surgery and pathology report

The patient underwent a 3D endoscopic nipple-sparing mastectomy with sentinel lymph node biopsy and immediate implant reconstruction. Intra-operative frozen section for both sentinel lymph node and sub-nipple biopsy were negative for metastases.

Her final histology showed a triple negative invasive ductal carcinoma with DCIS (T2N0M0), and she received adjuvant chemotherapy thereafter.

Post-operative outcomes

Her hospitalization was uneventful, and there were no immediate complications encountered. The patient was satisfied with her post-operative cosmesis when she was reviewed in outpatient clinic.

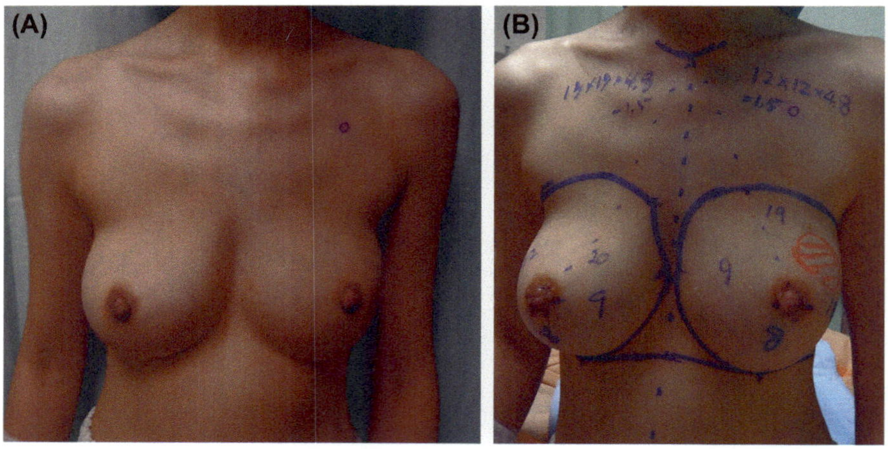

5.15A, B

Pre-operative front views showing pre-operative markings and location of tumor

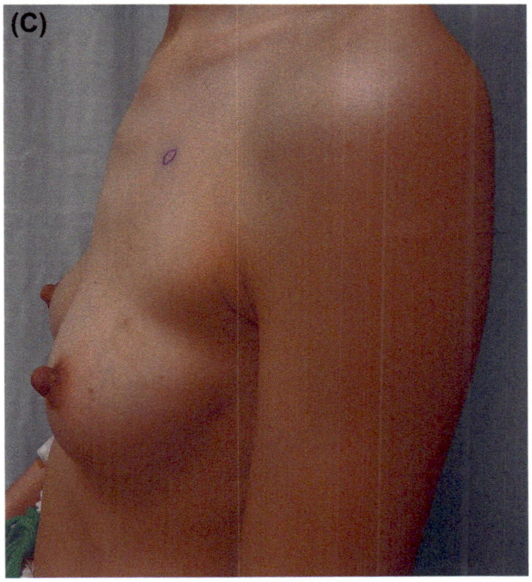

5.15C

Pre-operative lateral view

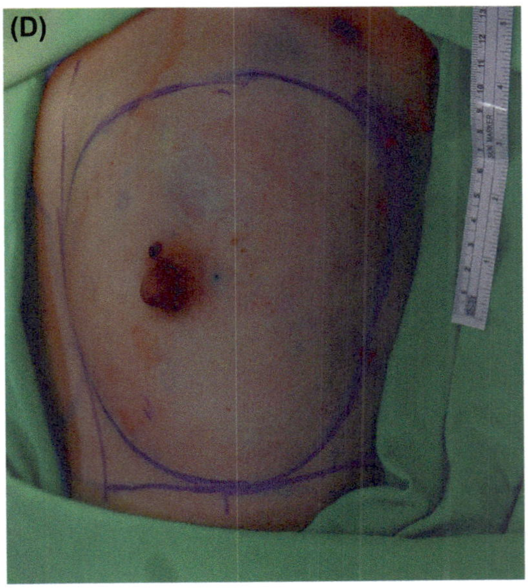

5.15D

On-table view showing the planned axillary incision

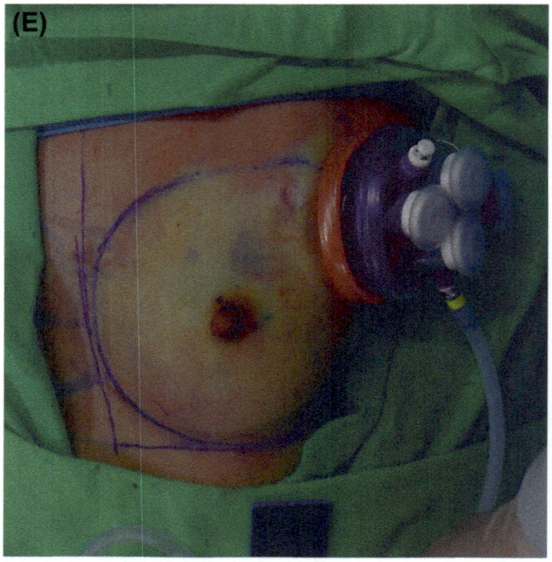

5.15E

Placement of the single port (Glove Port; Nelis Corporation, Gyeonggi-do, Korea) before commencement of mastectomy

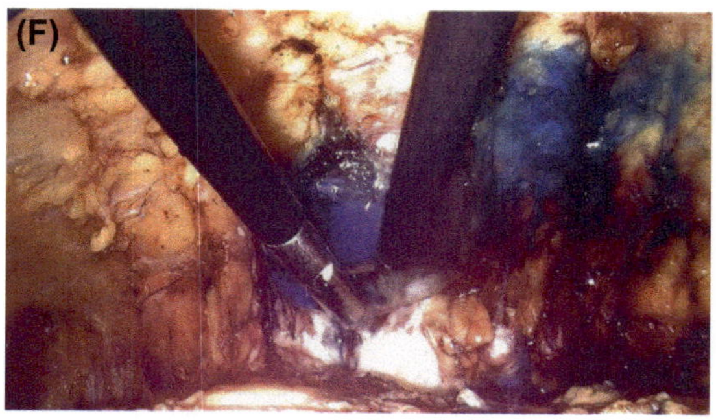

5.15F

Skin flap dissection and sub-nipple biopsies performed under 3D visualization

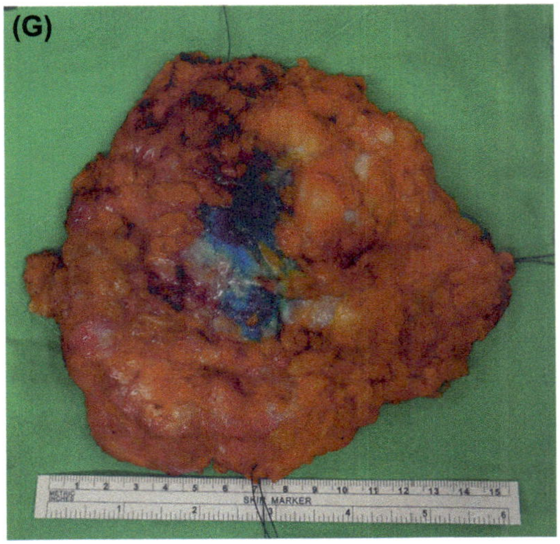

5.15G

Mastectomy specimen oriented with silk sutures

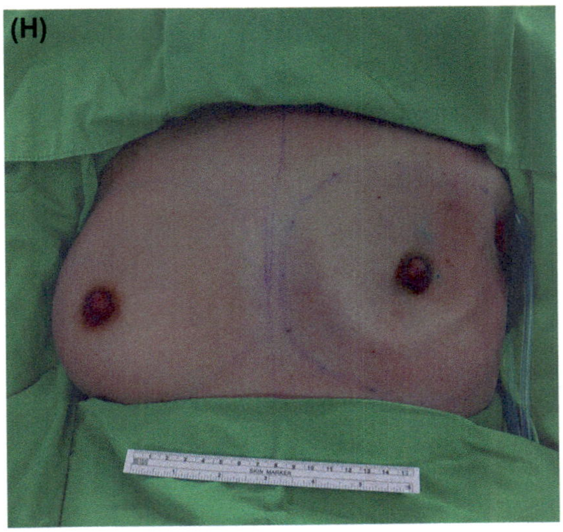

5.15H

On-table view after mastectomy

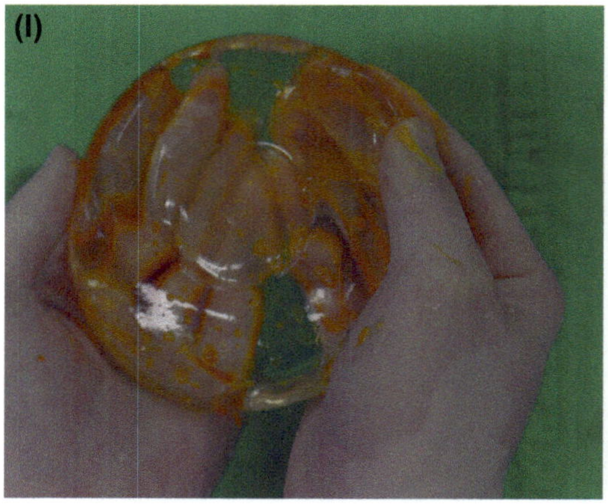

5.15I

Smooth implant of an appropriate volume chosen for immediate reconstruction

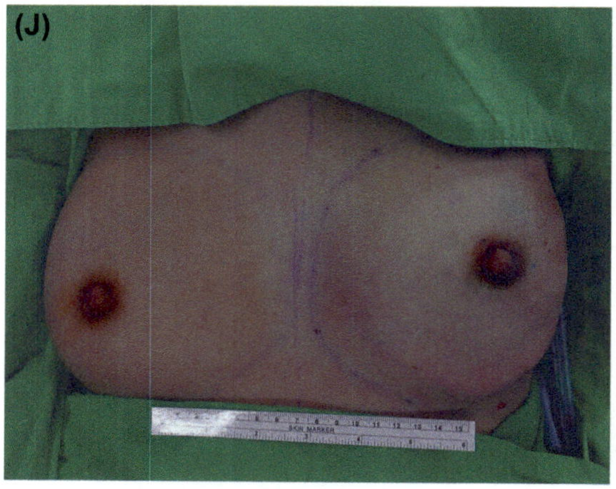

5.15J

Immediate on-table view after implant reconstruction

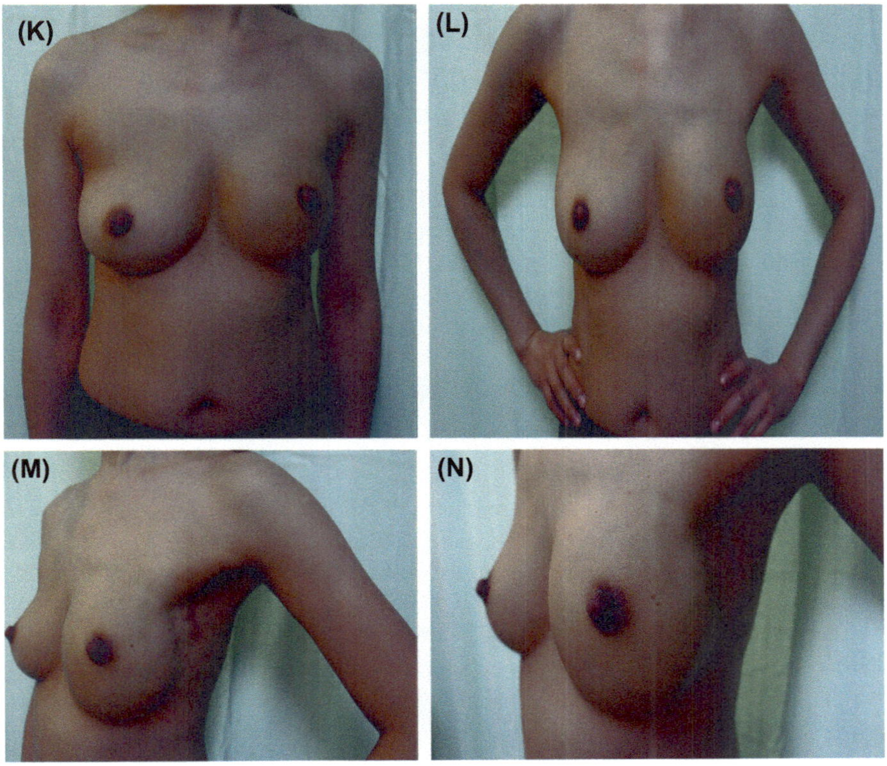

5.15K–N

3-month post-operative views showing well-hidden axillary scar and satisfactory aesthetic outcomes

Case 16: Bilateral three-dimensional (3D) endoscopic nipple-sparing mastectomy with immediate implant reconstruction – single incision, insufflation technique

Patient/demographics

This is a case of a 52-year-old lady with bilateral breast cancer. She initially presented a 7 cm right breast lump. Mammogram and ultrasound revealed another 2 cm suspicious lesion in her left breast. Core biopsy of the right breast lump returned as ductal carcinoma in situ while the left breast lump showed invasive ductal carcinoma. Patient opted for bilateral skin-sparing mastectomy and direct-to-implant reconstruction.

Her metastatic workup was otherwise negative.

Surgery and pathology report

Patient underwent a bilateral 3D endoscopic nipple-sparing mastectomy with sentinel lymph node biopsy and immediate implant reconstruction. Intra-operative frozen section for sentinel lymph node as well as sub-nipple biopsy was negative for metastases.

Her final histology showed a left breast invasive ductal carcinoma with ductal carcinoma in situ (T1bN0M0) and a right ductal carcinoma in situ with no invasive component (TisN0M0). She was recommended for 5 years of adjuvant endocrine therapy.

Post-operative outcomes

Her hospitalization was uneventful, and there were no immediate complications encountered. Patient was satisfied with her post-operative cosmesis when she was reviewed in outpatient clinic thereafter.

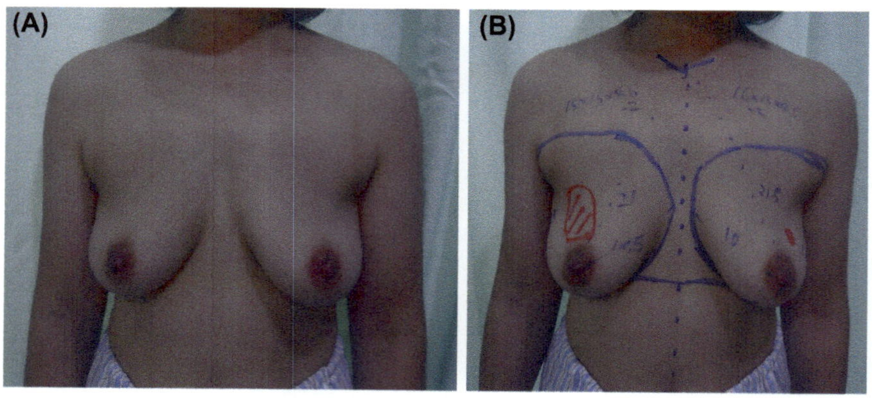

5.16A, 5.16B

Pre-operative front views showing pre-operative markings and location of tumor

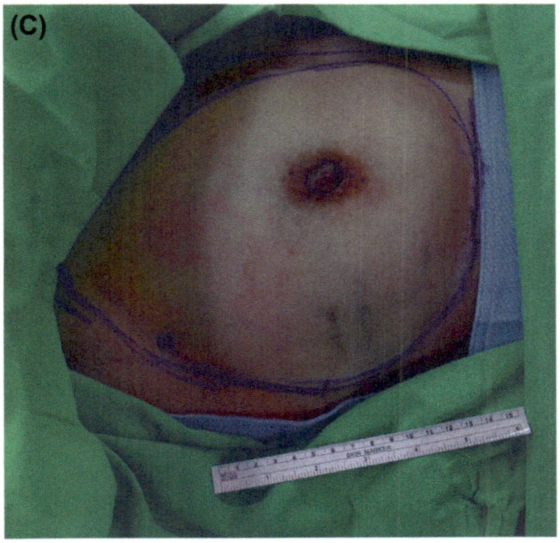

5.16C

On-table view showing the planned axillary incision

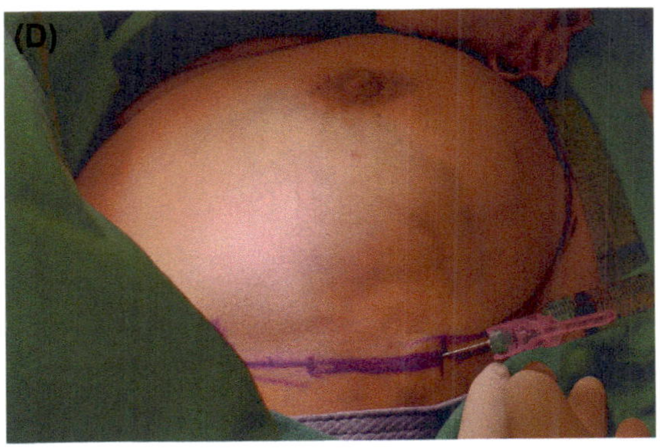

5.16D

Infiltration of local anesthetic before incision

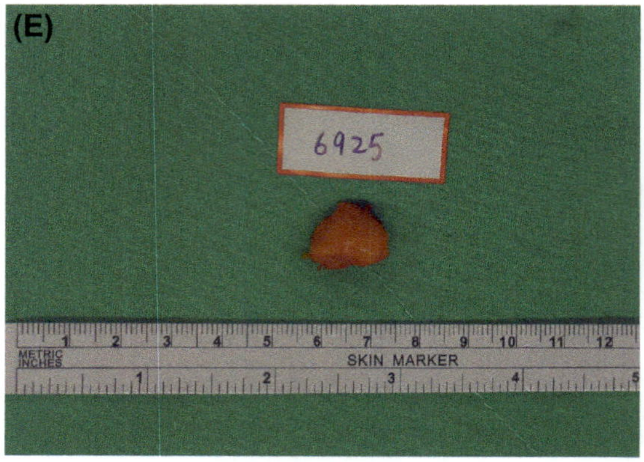

5.16E

Sentinel lymph node which was blue and hot, excised and sent for intra-operative frozen section analysis

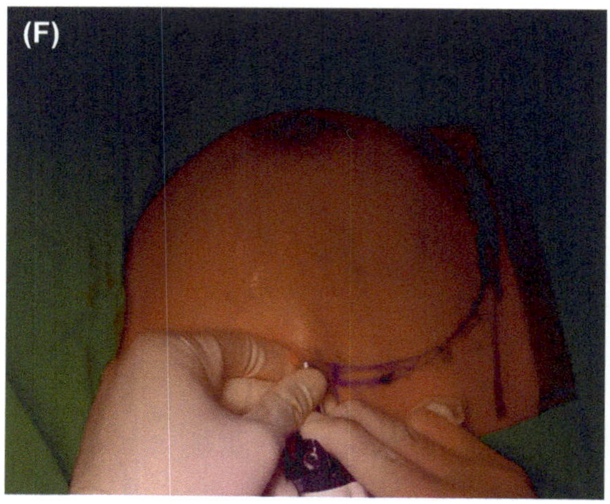

5.16F

Subcutaneous tunneling for subsequent skin flap dissection

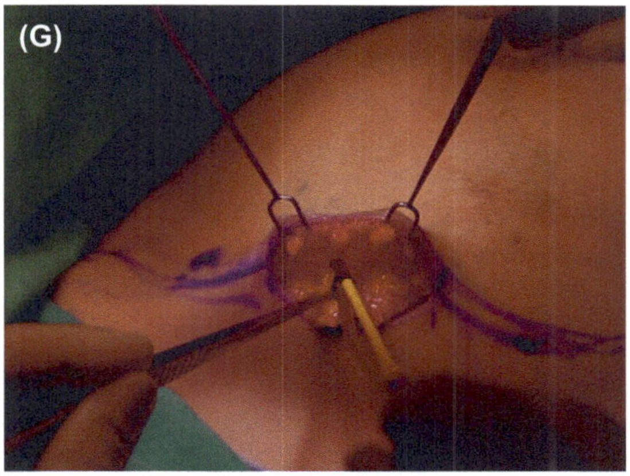

5.16G

Creation of working space before placement of single port

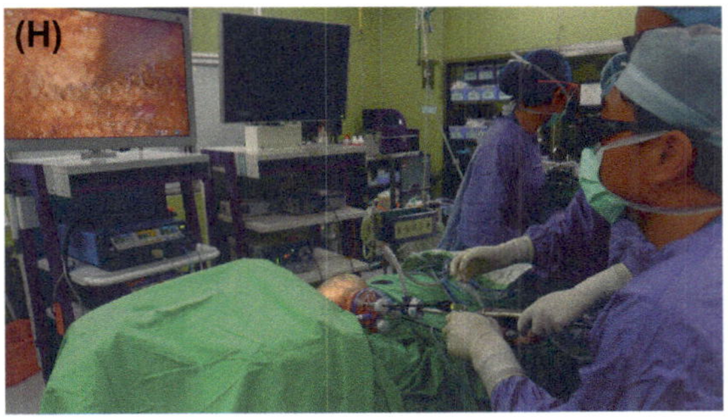

5.16H

Placement of the single port (Glove Port; Nelis Corporation, Gyeonggi-do, Korea) and intra-operative layout demonstrating the position of surgeon, first assistant, patient and endoscopic system

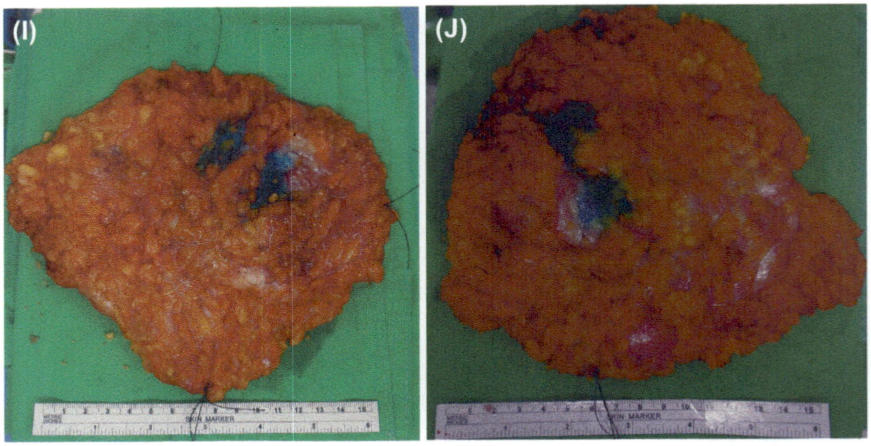

5.16I,J

Bilateral mastectomy specimens removed in entirety and oriented with silk sutures

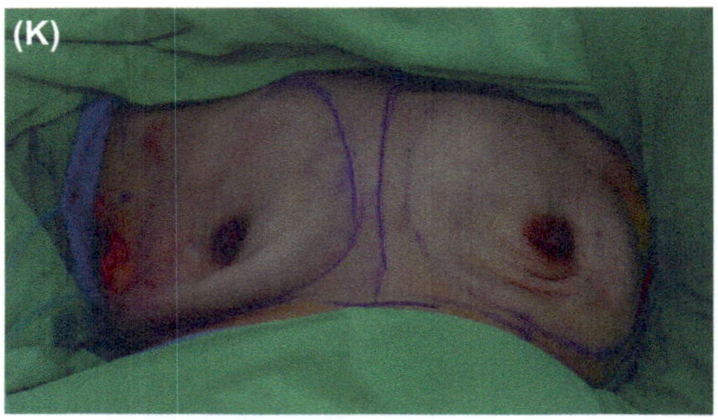

5.16K

Immediate on-table view after mastectomy

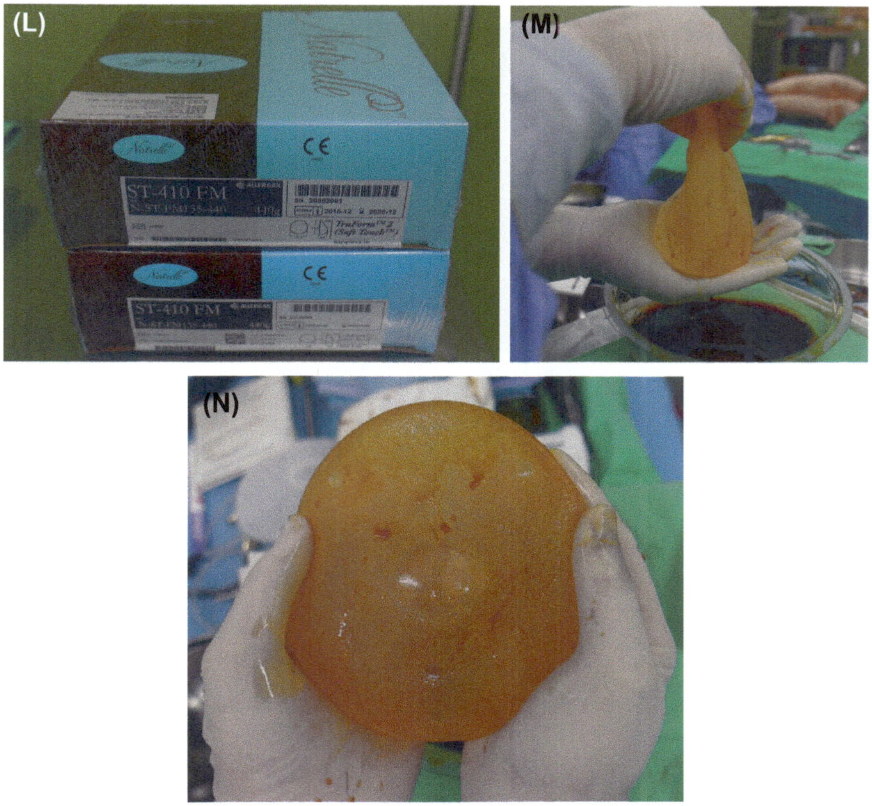

5.16L,M,N

Anatomical implant of an appropriate volume and size chosen for immediate reconstruction

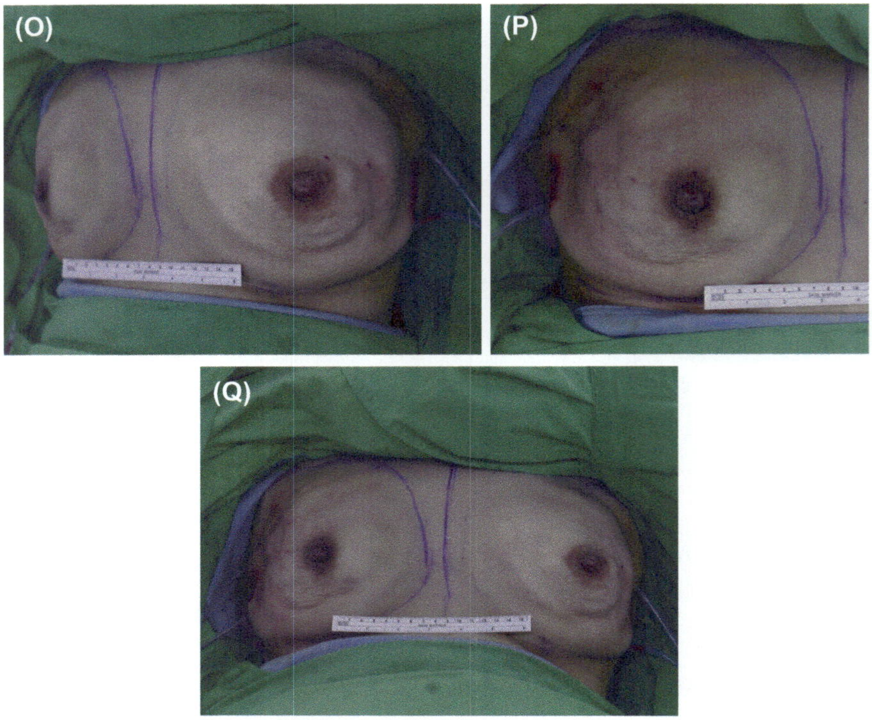

5.16O–Q

Immediate on-table views after implant reconstruction

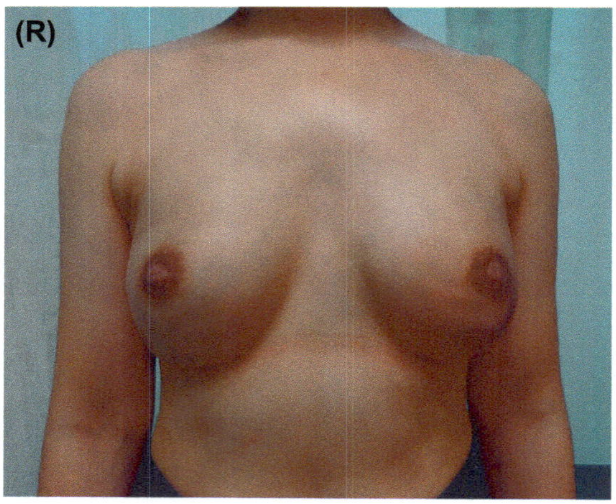

5.16R

3-month post-operative front view showing well-hidden incisions and satisfactory aesthetic outcomes

Discussion

Conventional endoscopic nipple-sparing mastectomy (E-NSM) techniques (Fukuma, 2006; Sakamoto et al., 2010) usually involve two separate small incisions, as demonstrated in Case 9. First, one incision is created over the axilla for axillary staging procedure and subsequently followed by endoscopic vein retractor harvesting, dissection, and separation of breast parenchyma from pectoralis muscle fascia. After complete dissection at the posterior aspect, a small peri-areolar wound is then created for dissection of septa between the breast parenchyma and skin flap. Mastectomy specimen is removed from either the peri-areolar or axillary incision. The resulting scar will normally be fairly inconspicuous, as they are hidden in the axilla or peri-areolar region. However, one of the commonly seen complications resulting from the peri-areolar incision would be NAC ischemia or necrosis which can be devastating, especially in cases of implant reconstruction whereby any secondary infection could be disastrous leading to possible implant removal. To reduce the risk of NAC ischemia/necrosis, the authors developed a new technique, which was demonstrated in Cases 8, 10 and 11 (Lai et al., 2018). This new technique utilized a single axillary incision which has demonstrated improved outcome in terms of NAC ischemia or necrosis in the authors' institution. To prevent surgical margin involvement and inadequate tumour resection, patient selection for single axillary-incision hybrid E-NSM is favoured in patients with tumours located in the upper outer quadrant and at an adequate distance from the skin. This technique may not be suitable in large and ptotic breast, as a single incision over IMF is a better choice for these patients whereby the scar is normally well hidden in the IMF. However, in small to medium-sized breast, scar in IMF will be more prominent than one placed in the axillary region. Hence, the authors would recommend a single axillary-incision endoscopic hybrid technique NSM for women diagnosed with early-stage, clinically node-negative breast cancer indicated for mastectomy, with small to medium-sized breast and minimal ptosis. A new technique modification of endoscopic nipple-sparing mastectomy using three-dimensional (3D) endoscopic system is now the preferred method in the authors' institutions, as the strength of this innovative surgical technique lies in the fact that it is safe and associated with good aesthetic outcomes as well as satisfactory operative time (Lai et al., 2016; Lai et al., 2019). It also addresses the technical difficulty in conventional two-dimensional (2D) E-NSM and compares favourably to robotic nipple-sparing mastectomy, R-NSM, in terms of cost.

References

Fukuma, E. (2006). Endoscopic breast surgery for breast cancer. *Nihon Geka Gakkai zasshi, 107*(2), 64–68.

Lai, H. W., et al. (2019). Single-port 3-dimensional Videoscope-assisted Endoscopic Nipple-sparing Mastectomy in the Management of Breast Cancer. *Plastic and Reconstructive Surgery.* https://doi.org/10.1097/GOX.0000000000002367. https://journals.lww.com/prsgo/toc/9000/00000.

Lai, H. W., Chen, S. T., Chen, D. R., Chen, S. L., Chang, T. W., Kuo, S. J., Kuo, Y. L., Hung, C. S., et al. (2016). Current Trends in and Indications for Endoscopy-Assisted Breast Surgery for Breast Cancer: Results from a Six-Year Study Conducted by the Taiwan Endoscopic Breast Surgery Cooperative Group. *PLoS One, 11*(3), e0150310. https://doi.org/10.1371/journal.pone.0150310. https://www.ncbi.nlm.nih.gov/pubmed/26950469. eCollection 2016. PMID:26950469.

Lai, H. W., Lin, S. L., Chen, S. T., Kuok, K. M., Chen, S. L., Lin, Y. L., et al. (2018). Single-axillary-incision endoscopic-assisted hybrid technique for nipple-sparing mastectomy: Technique, preliminary results, and patient-reported cosmetic outcome from preliminary 50 procedures. *Annals of Surgical Oncology, 25*(5), 1340−1349. https://doi.org/10.1245/s10434-018-6383-z.

Sakamoto, N., Fukuma, E., Higa, K., Ozaki, S., Sakamoto, M., Abe, S., et al. (2010). Early results of an endoscopic nipple-sparing mastectomy for breast cancer. *Indian Journal of Surgical Oncology, 1*(3), 232−239. https://doi.org/10.1007/s13193-011-0057-7.

CHAPTER 6

Endoscopic mastectomy with immediate transverse rectus abdominis flap reconstruction

Description of technique

Pre-operative marking and positioning

Pre-operative marking was done with the patient in standing and supine position. After induction of general anaesthesia, the patient was then placed in the supine position and ipsilateral arm abducted to 90 degrees to avoid affecting the operative procedure. Endoscopic video monitors (Olympus Optical Co., Tokyo, Japan) were set up on both sides of the patient's head to allow both the surgeon and assistant to view the monitor. An oblique-ended rigid endoscope measuring 5 mm in diameter with a viewing angle of 30 degrees was used in all procedures.

Axillary staging procedure

In patients for whom sentinel lymph node biopsy (SLNB) is indicated, a small amount (2−3 mCi) of radioisotope Tc99m was injected intradermally at the site of the tumour before operation (either on the day or 1 day prior).

After induction of general anaesthesia, 3 mL of 1% methylene blue (Merck, Darmstadt, Germany) was injected into the breast parenchyma in equally divided aliquots at five positions surrounding the hemisphere of the tumour facing the ipsilateral axilla. The breast tissue from the tumour to the axilla was then gently massaged for 5−10 minutes. Within 20−30 minutes after injection of the blue dye, a handheld gamma probe (Navigator; USSC, Norwalk, CT) was used to identify the hot spots and the location of the hottest nodes was then marked. An approximately 3-cm oblique axillary incision was then made close to the hottest nodes, and SLNB was then performed. Fresh frozen section was performed as indicated. If SLN was positive for metastases, a complete axillary lymph node dissection up to level II was performed.

Dissection of breast parenchyma off pectoralis major fascia

After completion of axillary staging procedure, dissection was carried out to the lateral border of the pectoralis major muscle. The margin between pectoralis muscle

Minimally Invasive (Endoscopic & Robotic) Breast Surgery. https://doi.org/10.1016/B978-0-323-73405-9.00006-6

and breast parenchyma was clearly identified. An endoscopic Ultra Retractor (Johnson & Johnson KK or Karl Storz) vein harvester was used for the dissection pectoral muscle fascia off posterior portion of breast parenchyma. The penetrating vessels were coagulated and cut with bipolar scissors (PowerStar, Johnson & Johnson KK) or a harmonic scalpel to ensure adequate haemostasis and therefore better visual clarity. Counter traction was applied by retracting surrounding tissue with the Ultra Retractor under endoscopic guidance to create a sufficient working space, and a suction tube can be used to evacuate mist and smoke.

Tunnelling and development of skin flap

After completion of the axillary staging procedure, a semi-circular peri-areolar skin incision or a single axillary incision was made (depending on surgeon's preference) as previously described. A physiological saline solution containing lidocaine 0.05% and epinephrine 1:1,000,000 was injected subcutaneously into the whole breast to minimize bleeding. An approximately 3–5-mm-thick skin flap was created via tunnelling method using an optical bladeless trocar Xcel (Johnson & Johnson, Tokyo, Japan) under endoscopic guidance. Subsequently, the septa between the skin flap and parenchyma was dissected and taken off under endoscopic guidance using endoscissors, bipolar scissors, or a harmonic scalpel.

Mastectomy

Following adequate skin flap development, a sub-areolar biopsy and fresh frozen section analysis can be performed in a nipple-sparing mastectomy. If cancer cell invasion was found in the sub-areolar area, the entire nipple-areola complex was removed and conversion to a skin-sparing mastectomy was then performed. After completion of skin flap development as well as detaching the breast off the pectoralis major fascia, the entire breast specimen can be removed via the axillary or peri-areolar incisions.

Immediate pedicled transversus rectus abdominis myocutaneous flap reconstruction

Transversus rectus abdominis myocutaneous (TRAM) flap design used by the authors allowed for superior extension above the umbilicus to include more perforators thereby enhancing flap vascularity. Flap harvesting started from the superior incision with dissection down the subcutaneous tissue till the fascia was encountered. After separating the upper part of the flap from the rectus fascia, the patient was flexed to ensure the extent of the lower incision allowed for a tension-free closure. The dissection then continued with elevation of the flap in a lateral to medial fashion, until the lateral rectus perforators were seen within which the anterior rectus sheath is reached. Both the medial and lateral edges of the rectus sheath were identified and preserved. Over the superior aspect of the TRAM, the sheath was incised up to the costal margin. Inferiorly, the deep inferior epigastric vessels were routinely dissected and ligated at their origin. The rectus muscle was then transected at this level. Posteriorly, the rectus flap was lifted off the posterior rectus sheath up to the costal margin. With the flap fully elevated and free except for its pedicle on the superior epigastric vessels, it was partly de-epithelialized to assess for blood flow and viability. Excess flap tissue was excised and discarded as necessary. Moving on, the abdomen was undermined up to the xiphoid process and a subcutaneous tunnel of 4–5 cm widths connecting the mastectomy site was created to allow for subsequent reconstruction. Further de-epithelization of the flap was performed as necessary depending on the amount of skin that requires preservation. In cases of nipple-sparing mastectomy, the whole flap could be de-epithelized. Four suction drains were placed (two at the donor site and two at the mastectomy site).

Case 17: endoscopic nipple-sparing mastectomy with immediate pedicled transversus rectus abdominis myocutaneous flap reconstruction

Patient/demographics

This is a case of a 35-year-old lady who presented with two hard palpable lumps in her left breast. Both lumps were suspicious on mammographic and sonographic evaluations, and core biopsies for both lumps showed invasive ductal carcinoma which was hormone responsive.

Her metastatic workup was negative.

As this patient had a multicentric tumor, conservation was not suitable and she opted for a nipple-sparing mastectomy with immediate reconstruction. Option of autologous free-flap reconstruction was offered, but the patient was keen for a pedicled flap instead.

Surgery and pathology report

The patient underwent left endoscopic nipple-sparing mastectomy, sentinel lymph node biopsy, and immediate pedicled transversus rectus abdominis myocutaneous (TRAM) flap reconstruction.

Her pathology report showed a T2N0M0 stage 2A disease. She subsequently received adjuvant chemotherapy and endocrine therapy for 5 years.

Post-operative outcomes

The patient was discharged well 2 days after operation. Her post-operative recovery was complicated with per-areolar wound breakdown and secondary infection approximately 2 weeks after operation.

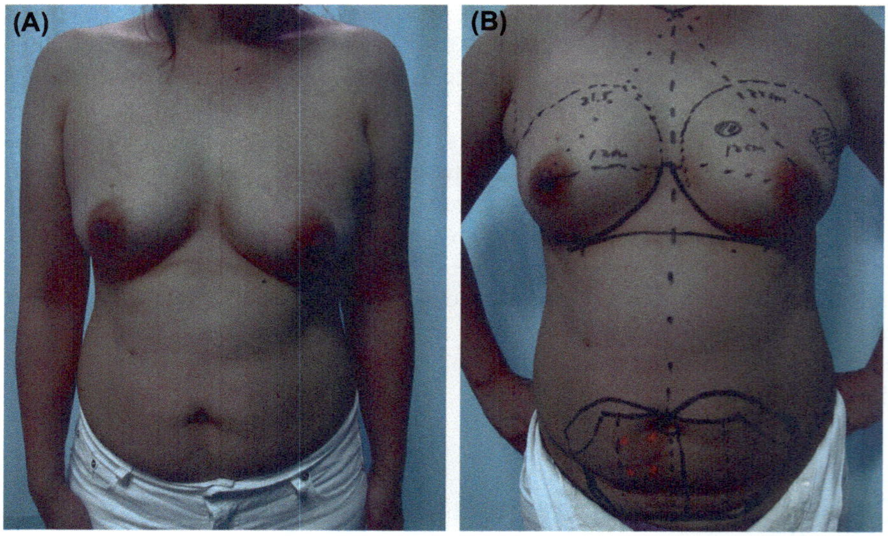

6.17A, B

Pre-operative front views showing pre-operative markings and location of tumor.

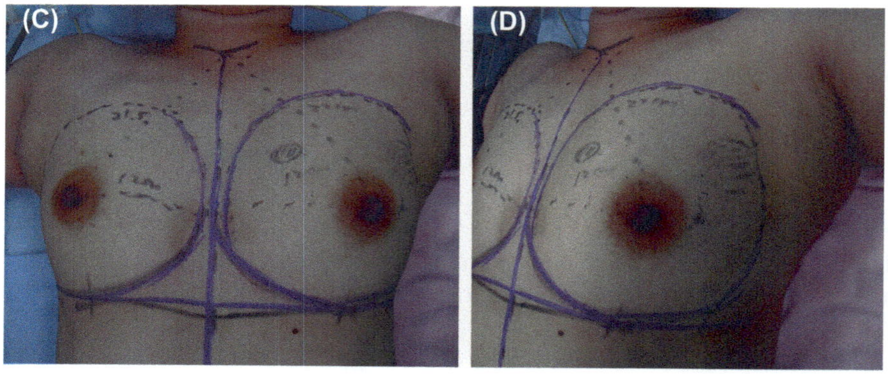

6.17C, D

On-table markings showing location of tumor and planned axillary incision.

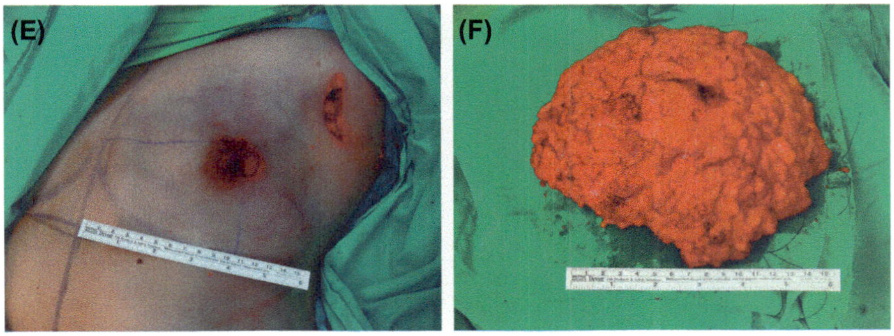

6.17E, F

Immediate on-table view after mastectomy with specimen extracted via axillary incision.

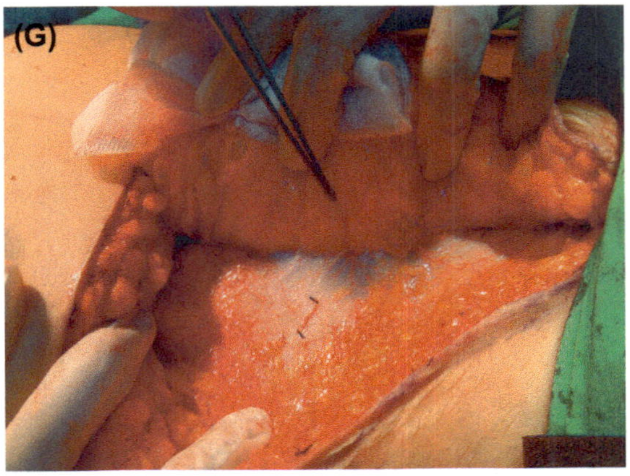

6.17G

Perforator vessels arising from the rectus sheath as shown earlier.

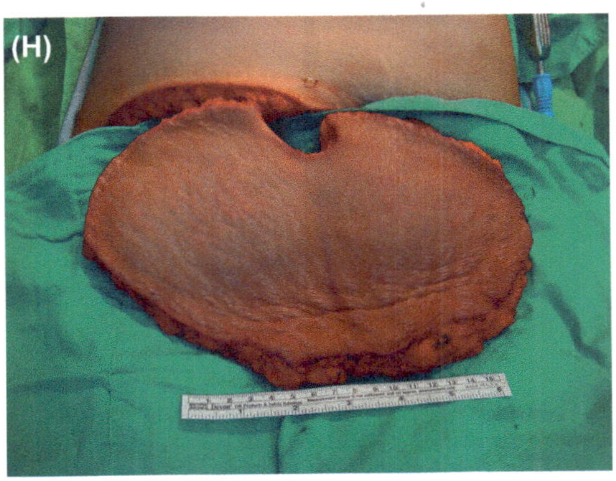

6.17H

TRAM flap completely raised.

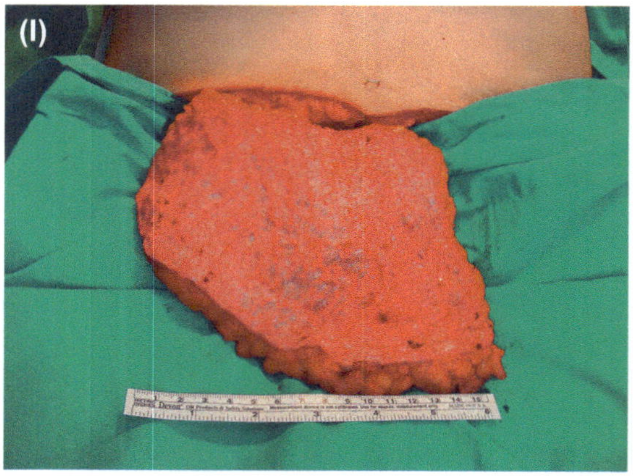

6.17I

Excision of zone 4 and partial zone 3 with flap completely de-epithelized before reconstruction.

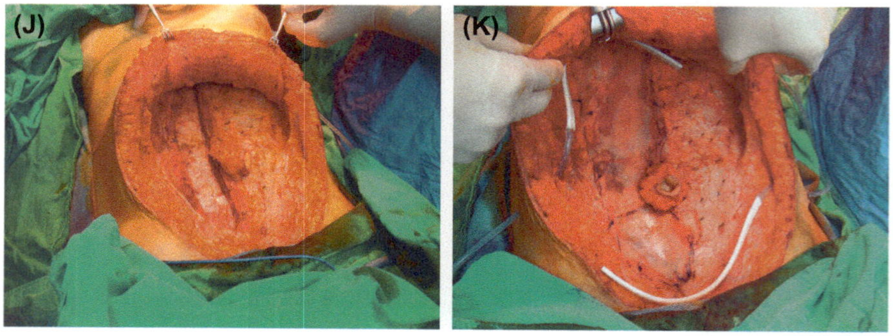

6.17J, K

Contralateral pedicled TRAM flap fully mobilized and tunneled into left breast mastectomy cavity. Defect repaired with mesh placement and two drains placed in the donor site thereafter.

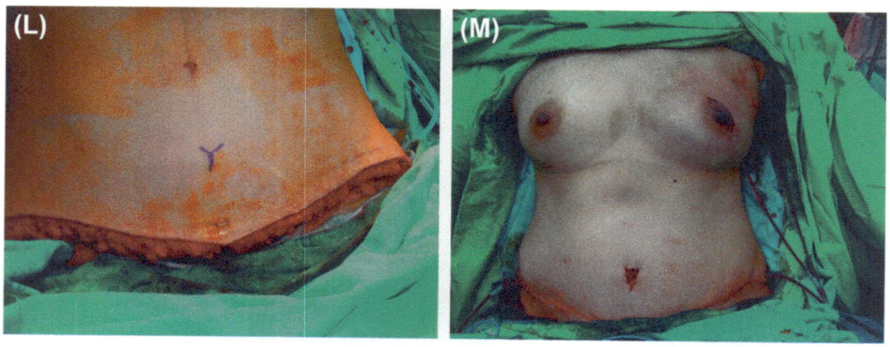

6.17L, M

Neo-umbilicus location as shown in (L) and final post-operative view shown in (m).

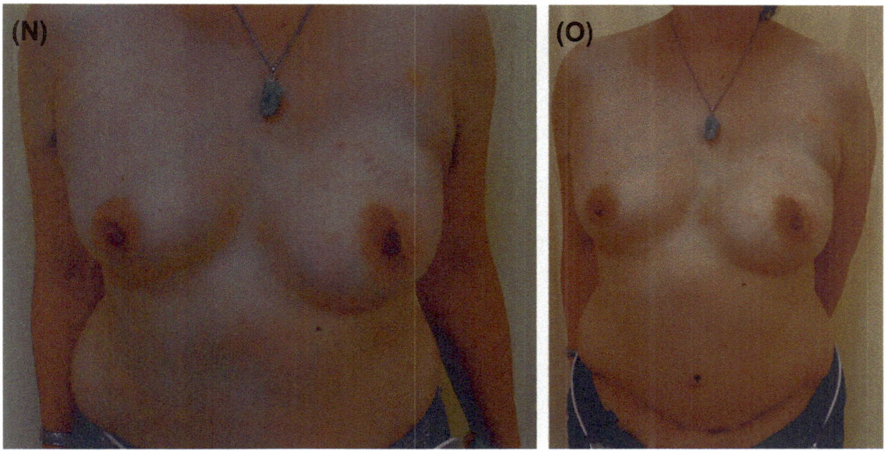

6.17N,

o4 years post-operative view. Hypopigmented scar seen over left peri-areolar wound attiributed to partial nipple areolar complex ischemia/necrosis.

Discussion

Breast reconstruction following endoscopy-assisted total mastectomy normally involves the use of tissue expanders (TE) or gel-filled implants. Endoscopic-assisted nipple- or skin-sparing mastectomy combined with immediate breast reconstruction with pedicled TRAM flap has been shown to be a safe procedure and results in good cosmetic outcome in patients with early-stage breast cancer. Reconstruction with a pedicled TRAM flap, however, is technically demanding, results in additional scarring over the lower abdomen, and is associated with prolonged operative time (Andrades et al., 2008). When TRAM flap reconstruction is planned, patients should be informed of the risk of donor site morbidities and potential flap loss. The authors believe that this procedure is particularly beneficial for patients with large or ptotic breasts in which sub-pectoral TE/implant-based reconstruction often results in suboptimal cosmetic outcome (Lai et al., 2015). Obese patients with loose abdominal skin can also benefit from the abdominoplasty. Another group of patients might be those who will require post-operative radiotherapy, as the risks of capsular contracture for implant-based reconstruction post-radiotherapy is a concern. An autologous TRAM flap in this case would be fairly resistant to volume loss secondary to radiotherapy (Carlson et al., 2008).

References

Andrades, P., Fix, R. J., Danilla, S., Howell, R. E., 3rd, Campbell, W. J., De la Torre, J., et al. (2008). Ischemic complications in pedicle, free, and muscle sparing transverse rectus abdominis myocutaneous flaps for breast reconstruction. *Annals of Plastic Surgery.* https://doi.org/10.1097/SAP.0b013e31816fc372.

Carlson, G. W., Page, A. L., Peters, K., Ashinoff, R., Schaefer, T., & Losken, A. (2008). Effects of radiation therapy on pedicled transverse rectus abdominis myocutaneous flap breast reconstruction. *Annals of Plastic Surgery.* https://doi.org/10.1097/SAP.0b013e31815b6ced.

Lai, H. W., Wu, H. S., Chuang, K. L., Chen, D. R., Chang, T. W., Kuo, S. J., et al. (2015). Endoscopy-assisted total mastectomy followed by immediate pedicled transverse rectus abdominis musculocutaneous (TRAM) flap reconstruction: Preliminary results of 48 patients. *Surgical Innovation.* https://doi.org/10.1177/1553350614546003.

CHAPTER

Endoscopic mastectomy with immediate latissimus dorsi flap reconstruction

7

Description of technique

Pre-operative marking and positioning

Pre-operative marking was done with the patient in standing and supine position. After induction of general anaesthesia, the patient was then placed in the supine position and ipsilateral arm abducted to 90 degrees to avoid affecting the operative procedure. Endoscopic video monitors (Olympus Optical Co., Tokyo, Japan) were set up on both sides of the patient's head to allow both the surgeon and assistant to view the monitor. An oblique-ended rigid endoscope measuring 5 mm in diameter with a viewing angle of 30 degrees was used in all procedures.

Axillary staging procedure

In patients for whom sentinel lymph node biopsy (SLNB) is indicated, a small amount (2–3 mCi) of radioisotope Tc99m was injected intradermally at the site of the tumour before operation (either on the day or 1 day prior).

After induction of general anaesthesia, 3 mL of 1% methylene blue (Merck, Darmstadt, Germany) was injected into the breast parenchyma in equally divided aliquots at five positions surrounding the hemisphere of the tumour facing the ipsilateral axilla. The breast tissue from the tumour to the axilla was then gently massaged for 5–10 minutes. Within 20–30 minutes after injection of the blue dye, a handheld gamma probe (Navigator; USSC, Norwalk, CT) was used to identify the hot spots, and the location of the hottest nodes was then marked. An approximately 3-cm oblique axillary incision was then made close to the hottest nodes, and SLNB was then performed. Fresh frozen section was performed as indicated. If SLN was positive for metastases, a complete axillary lymph node dissection up to level II was performed.

Dissection of breast parenchyma off pectoralis major fascia

After completion of axillary staging procedure, dissection was carried out to the lateral border of the pectoralis major muscle. The margin between pectoralis muscle and breast parenchyma was clearly identified. An endoscopic Ultra Retractor

Minimally Invasive (Endoscopic & Robotic) Breast Surgery. https://doi.org/10.1016/B978-0-323-73405-9.00007-8

(Johnson & Johnson KK or Karl Storz) vein harvester was used for the dissection pectoral muscle fascia off posterior portion of breast parenchyma. The penetrating vessels were coagulated and cut with bipolar scissors (PowerStar, Johnson & Johnson KK) or a harmonic scalpel to ensure adequate haemostasis and therefore better visual clarity. Counter traction was applied by retracting surrounding tissue with the Ultra Retractor under endoscopic guidance to create a sufficient working space, and a suction tube can be used to evacuate mist and smoke.

Tunnelling and development of skin flap

After completion of the axillary staging procedure, a physiological saline solution containing lidocaine 0.05% and epinephrine 1:1,000,000 was injected subcutaneously into the whole breast to minimize bleeding. An approximately 3—5-mm-thick skin flap was created via tunnelling method using an optical bladeless trocar Xcel (Johnson & Johnson, Tokyo, Japan) under endoscopic guidance. Subsequently, the septa between the skin flap and parenchyma was dissected and taken off under endoscopic guidance using endoscissors, bipolar scissors, or a harmonic scalpel.

Mastectomy

Following adequate skin flap development, a sub-areolar biopsy and fresh frozen section analysis can be performed in a nipple-sparing mastectomy. If cancer cell invasion was found in the sub-areolar area, the entire nipple-areola complex was removed and conversion to a skin-sparing mastectomy was then performed. After completion of skin flap development as well as detaching the breast off the pectoralis major fascia, the entire breast specimen can be removed via the axillary incision.

Immediate pedicled latissimus dorsi flap reconstruction

Following removal of the specimen and adequate haemostasis, copious irrigation of the mastectomy pocket was performed. Subsequently, the thoracodorsal pedicle was identified and marked with a vessel loop to prevent injury during the flap harvest. Patient was then shifted to the lateral decubitus position. Dissection started along the under surface of the latissimus dorsi (LD) muscle with endoscopic Ultra Retractor (Johnson & Johnson KK or Karl Storz) vein harvester and Harmonic scalpel. Blood vessels encountered were carefully dissected, coagulated and cut. As the dissection through the under surface of the muscle to the borders was completed, further dissection over the superficial surface of the muscle ensued. The muscle was disconnected from the infero-posterior and scapular border. Afterwards, the pedicled LD flap was exteriorized from the axilla wound. Reconstruction of the mastectomy defect was performed with the patient turned back to a supine position. Fixation of the flap to all quadrants was performed with assistance from a handle light retractor to ensure full coverage of the defect. Care must be taken to ensure the correct axis of the vascular pedicle to prevent torsion of the blood supply. Drains were then placed both in the donor site as well as mastectomy cavity.

Case 18: endoscopic nipple-sparing mastectomy with immediate pedicled latissimus dorsi flap reconstruction

Patient/demographics

This is a case of a 48-year-old lady who presented with a left breast lump which was suspicious looking on imaging. Core biopsies for the lumps showed invasive ductal carcinoma which was hormone responsive. Her metastatic workup was negative. As the tumor was 6 cm on presentation, the patient was counseled for neoadjuvant chemotherapy which was completed uneventfully. There was only partial response, and the patient opted for a nipple-sparing mastectomy with pedicled latissimus dorsi (LD) flap reconstruction.

Surgery and pathology report

The patient underwent left endoscopic nipple-sparing mastectomy, sentinel lymph node biopsy, and immediate pedicled LD flap reconstruction. Sentinel lymph node biopsy was negative and her pathology report showed a ypT2N0M0 disease. She subsequently received adjuvant endocrine therapy without disease recurrence.

Post-operative outcomes

The patient was discharged well 4 days after operation. Her post-operative recovery was uneventful, and the review in the outpatient clinic reported satisfactory cosmesis.

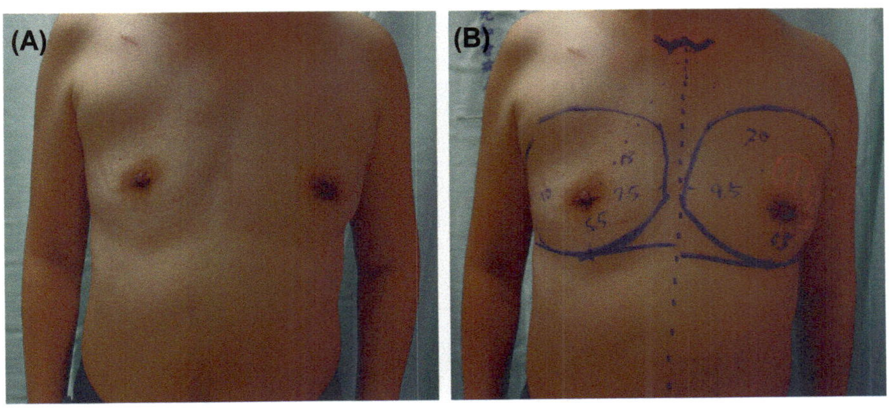

7.18A, B

Pre-operative front views showing pre-operative markings and location of tumor.

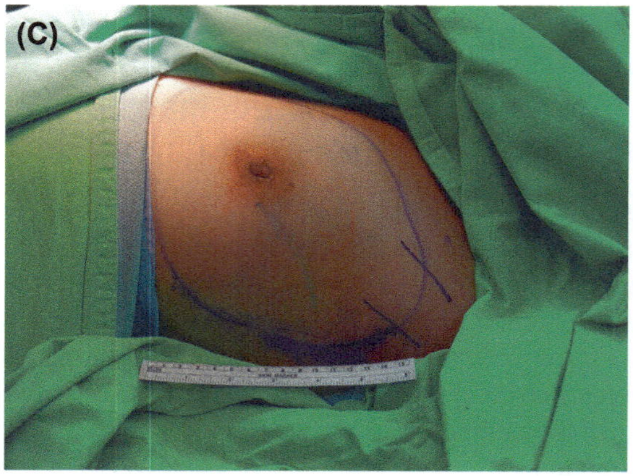

7.18C

On-table markings showing location of planned axillary incision.

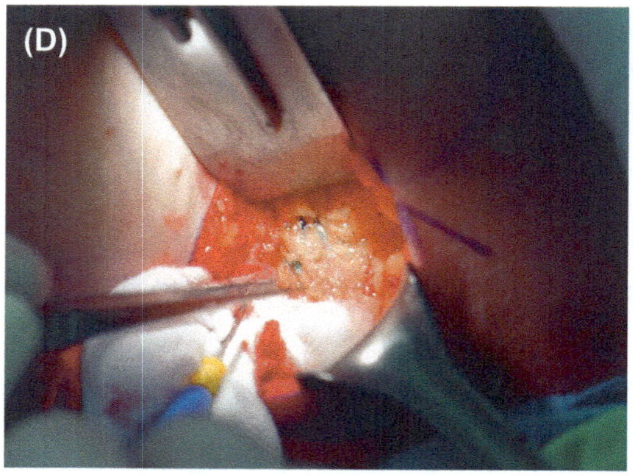

7.18D

Sentinel lymph node identified.

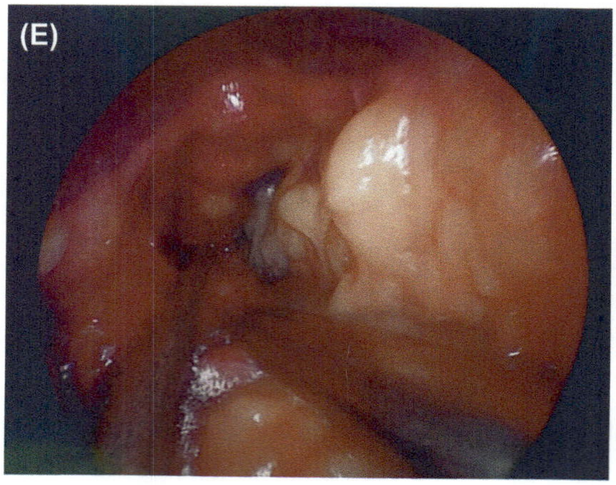

7.18E

Endoscopic view showing dissection of septa between skin and breast parenchyma.

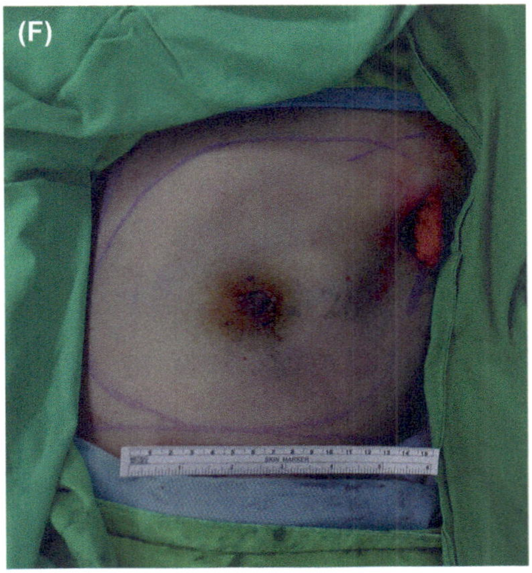

7.18F

Immediate on-table view after mastectomy with specimen extracted via axillary incision.

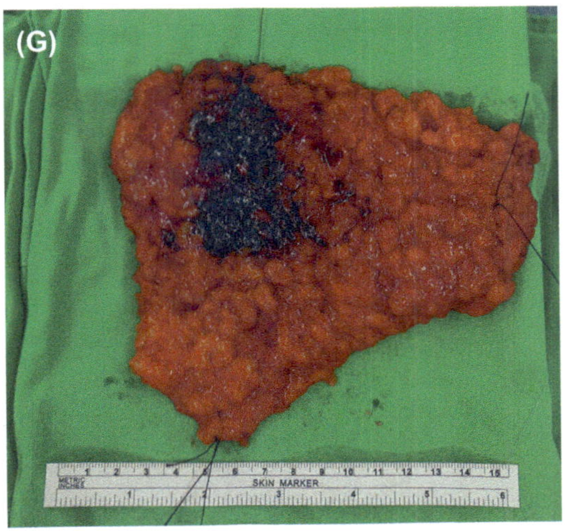

7.18G

Mastectomy specimen intact and oriented.

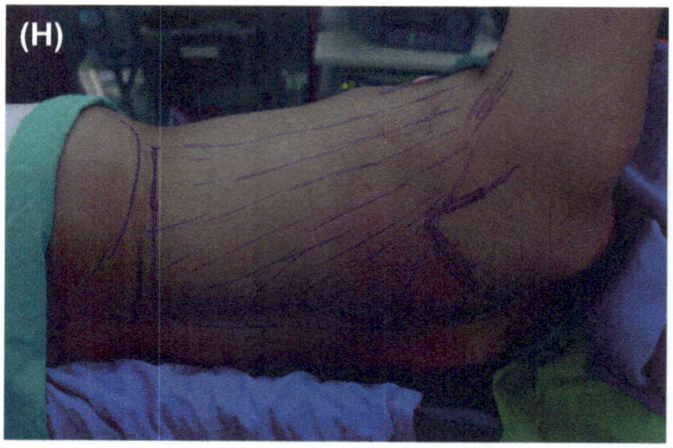

7.18H

Landmark markings for LD flap and extent of dissection.

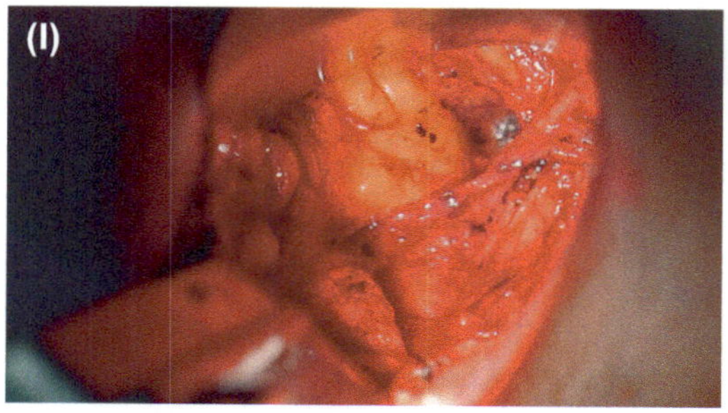

7.18I

Thoracodorsal bundle identified clearly and slung with vessel loop before flap harvest.

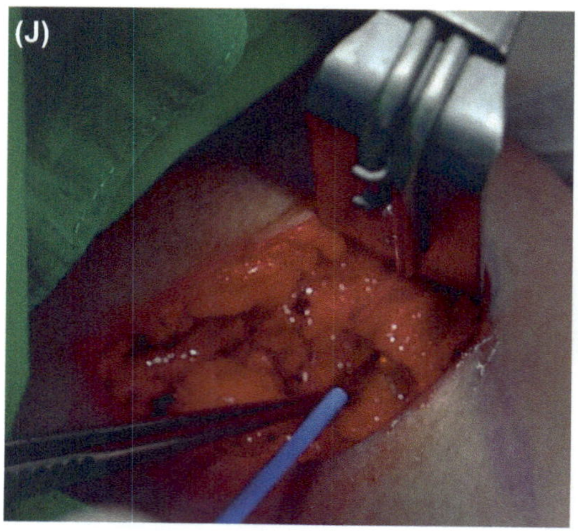

7.18J

Dissection and flap harvest from latissimus dorsi border via axillary incision.

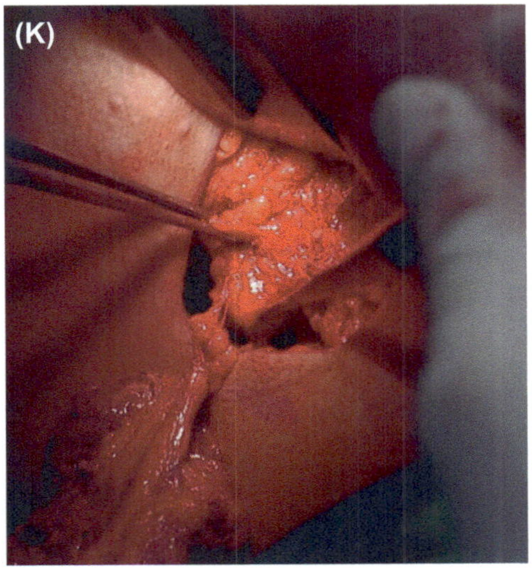

7.18K

Care taken not to injure thoracodorsal bundle.

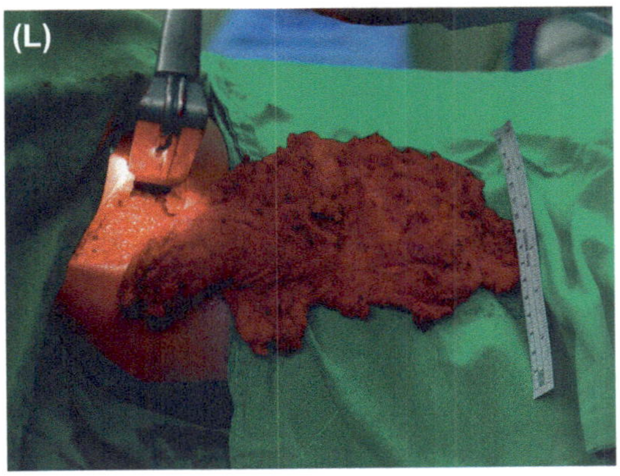

7.18L

Left pedicled LD flap exteriorized.

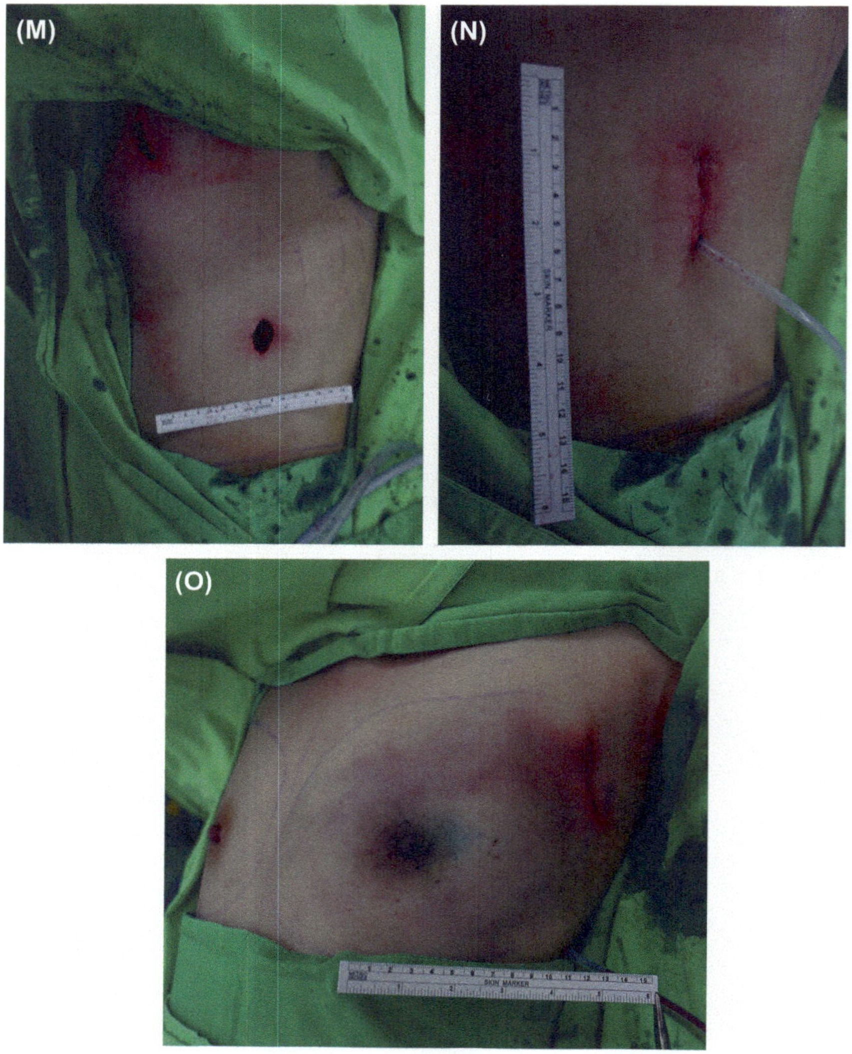

7.18M–O

Small axillary and midaxillary incision as shown in these immediate post-operative views.

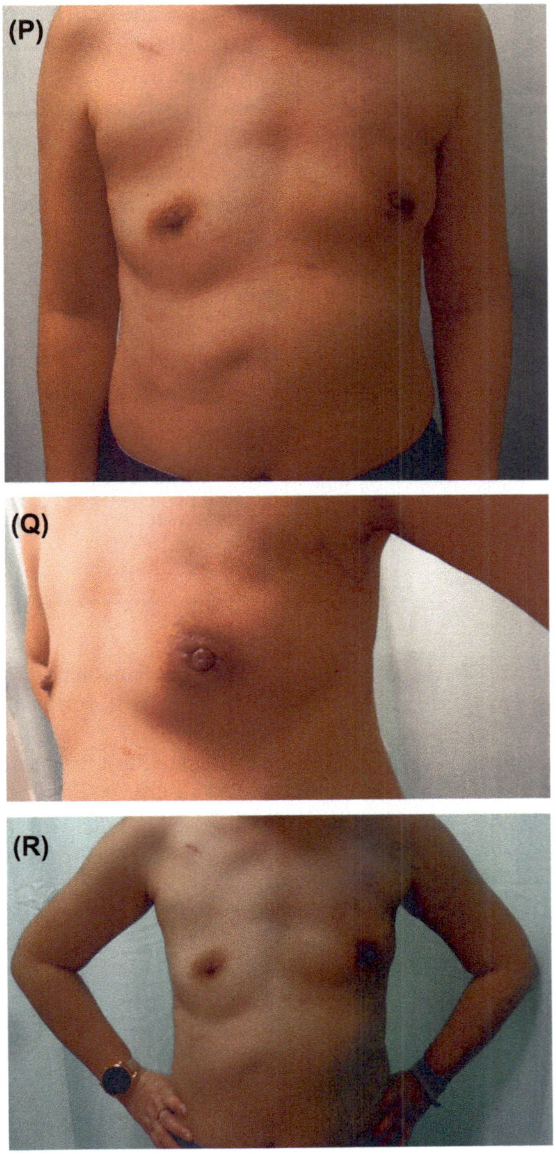

7.18P–R

1-year post-operative views showing well-healed and well-hidden scars.

Discussion

Latissimus dorsi flap, also known as the workhorse flap, has been widely used in a large variety of breast cancer defects from quadrantectomy to mastectomy. It can be used in either immediate or delayed reconstruction, alone or in combination with tissue expanders for a staged reconstruction with equally satisfactory outcome (Iglesias & Gonzalez-Chapa, 2013). Recent innovations and development in the workhorse flap include the advent of 'skinless' or 'scarless' approach via endoscopic-assisted harvest (Sood, Easow, Konopka, Panthaki, 2018). Endoscopic-assisted nipple- or skin-sparing mastectomy combined with immediate breast reconstruction with pedicled LD flap has the main advantage of a small and inconspicuous axillary wound. This is a major plus point compared to conventional LD flap harvest which involves leaving a long donor site incision. Other than cosmetically pleasing, avoidance of potential wound-related morbidities is also an important consideration. In addition, with the extent of skin incision taken out of the picture, one could potentially harvest the maximal amount of flap without worrying about wound closure. The potential downside of this procedure could be longer operation time in the learning phase (Missana & Pomel, 2007). In terms of patient selection, the authors believe that this reconstruction technique is most suitable for women with small to medium-sized breast with early breast cancer indicated for Nipple sparing mastectomy (NSM) while desiring an autologous breast reconstruction.

References

Iglesias, M., & Gonzalez-Chapa, D. R. (2013). Endoscopic latissimus dorsi muscle flap for breast reconstruction after skin-sparing total mastectomy: Report of 14 cases. *Aesthetic Plastic Surgery*. https://doi.org/10.1007/s00266-013-0131-3.

Missana, M. C., & Pomel, C. (2007). Endoscopic latissimus dorsi flap harvesting. *The American Journal of Surgery*. https://doi.org/10.1016/j.amjsurg.2006.10.029.

Sood, R., Easow, J. M., Konopka, G., & Panthaki, Z. J. (2018). Latissimus dorsi flap in breast reconstruction: Recent innovations in the workhorse flap. *Cancer Control*. https://doi.org/10.1177/1073274817744638.

PART

Robotic breast surgery

2

SECTION 1

Robotic breast surgery with no reconstruction

CHAPTER

Robotic mastectomy

8

Description of technique

Pre-operative marking and positioning

Pre-operative marking was done with the patient in standing and supine position. After induction of general anaesthesia, the patient was then placed in the supine position and ipsilateral arm abducted to 90 degrees to avoid affecting the operative procedure.

Axillary staging procedure

In patients for whom sentinel lymph node biopsy (SLNB) is indicated, a small amount (2−3 mCi) of radioisotope Tc99m was injected intradermally at the site of the tumour before operation (either on the day or 1 day prior).

After induction of general anaesthesia, 3 mL of 1% methylene blue (Merck, Darmstadt, Germany) was injected into the breast parenchyma in equally divided aliquots at five positions surrounding the hemisphere of the tumour facing the ipsilateral axilla. The breast tissue from the tumour to the axilla was then gently massaged for 5−10 minutes. Within 20−30 minutes after injection of the blue dye, a handheld gamma probe (Navigator; USSC, Norwalk, CT) was used to identify the hot spots and the location of the hottest nodes was then marked. An approximately 3−5 cm oblique axillary incision was then made close to the hottest nodes, and SLNB was then performed. Fresh frozen section was performed as indicated. If SLN was positive for metastases, a complete axillary lymph node dissection up to level II was performed.

Robotic docking and dissection

To create working space for placement of the single port (Glove Port; Nelis Corporation, Gyeonggi-do, Korea), a 3−4 cm subcutaneous flap was dissected with electro cautery under direct vision. The tunnelling technique as described in endoscopic mastectomy was then used to facilitate skin flap dissection and create space between the skin flap and the breast parenchyma. Once adequate dissection was achieved, the single port was then inserted through the axilla incision and carbon dioxide (CO_2) insufflation with air pressure kept at 8 mmHg was used to create space for mastectomy. The

Minimally Invasive (Endoscopic & Robotic) Breast Surgery. https://doi.org/10.1016/B978-0-323-73405-9.00008-X

ipsilateral shoulder was elevated to 30 degrees to prevent conflict between the operating table and docking of the robotic surgery system. The robotic side cart (da Vinci; Intuitive Surgical, Sunnyvale, CA, USA) was then positioned from the contralateral side, with the two robotic arms endoscope extending over the patient in proximity to the ports before the ports were docked to the robotic arms. Subsequently, the operation was then shifted to the da Vinci Si or Xi (Intuitive Surgical, Sunnyvale, CA, USA) robotic platform controlled by the operating surgeon at the console. The authors used a 30 degree 12-mm-diameter camera (Intuitive Surgical, Denzlingen, Germany) in the upper port to prevent collisions with other instruments. Dissection was carried out using an 8-mm monopolar scissors (Intuitive Surgical, Sunnyvale, CA, USA). Traction and counter-traction, along with maintaining exposure were carried out using an 8-mm ProGrasp forceps (Intuitive Surgical, Sunnyvale, CA, USA). The location of the scissors and the ProGrasp forceps could be changed inter-variably during the operation. Dissection was initiated from the superficial skin flaps by dissecting the septa between the skin flap and parenchyma created by the tunnelling technique with monopolar scissors. A sub-areolar biopsy and fresh frozen section analysis can be performed in a nipple-sparing mastectomy (NSM). If cancer cell invasion was found in the sub-areolar area, the entire nipple-areole complex (NAC) was removed and conversion to a skin-sparing mastectomy was then performed. After completion of the superficial skin flap dissection, dissection of the peripheral portion of the breast parenchyma was carried out subsequently. Posterior dissection was then performed by detaching the breast tissue from the pectoralis major muscle fascia with the perforator vessels clearly identified and secured. After completion of dissection, the entire breast specimen was removed through the axillary wound.

Case 19: robotic nipple-sparing mastectomy – single incision

Patient/demographics

The patient is a 40-year-old lady with newly diagnosed clinical stage IIA right breast invasive ductal carcinoma which was hormone responsive.

Pre-operative core biopsy report revealed an invasive ductal carcinoma with ductal carcinoma in situ. The patient opted for a mastectomy with no reconstruction, and she was also keen for a contralateral prophylactic mastectomy.

Her metastatic workup was negative.

Surgery and pathology report

The patient underwent bilateral robotic nipple-sparing mastectomy and right sentinel lymph node biopsy. The frozen section for sentinel lymph node biopsy and right sub-nipple biopsies were negative for metastases.

Her final histopathology reported a stage IIA T2N0M0 disease, and the patient subsequently received adjuvant chemotherapy and endocrine therapy for 5 years.

Post-operative outcomes

The patient was discharged after 2 days, and there were no immediate complications. She was satisfied with her post-operative cosmesis.

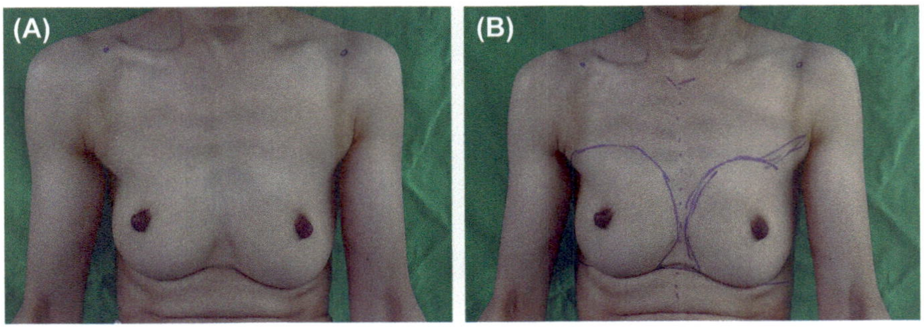

8.19A, B

Pre-operative front views showing pre-operative markings.

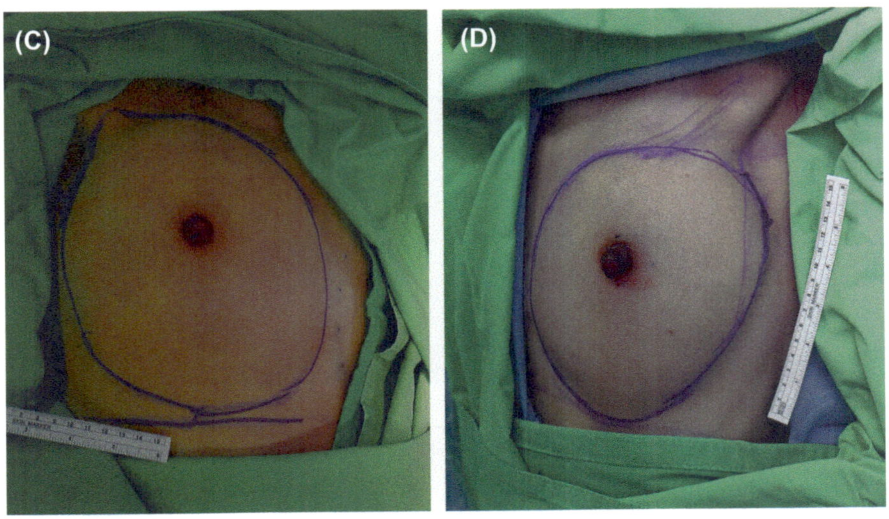

8.19C, D

On-table markings showing extent of planned dissection and placement of axillary incision.

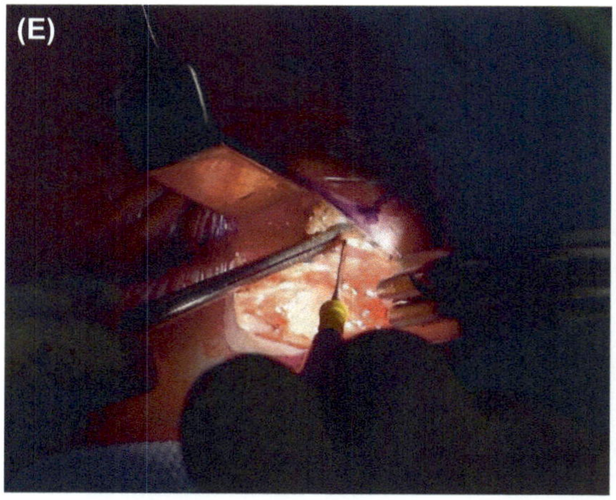

8.19E

Sentinel lymph node biopsy performed via axillary incision.

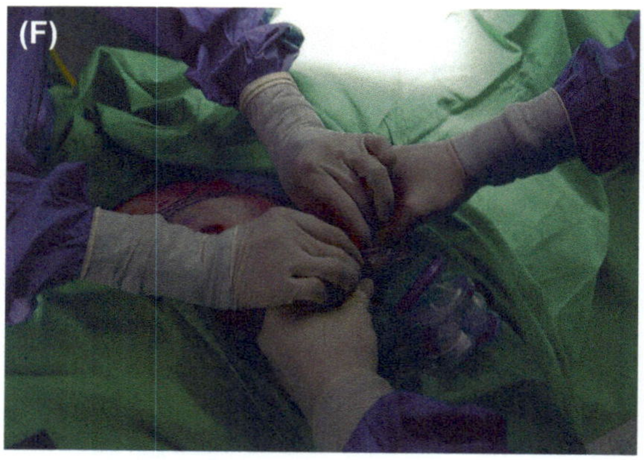

8.19F

Single port (Glove Port; Nelis Corporation, Gyeonggi-do, Korea) used in single axillary incision robotic mastectomy.

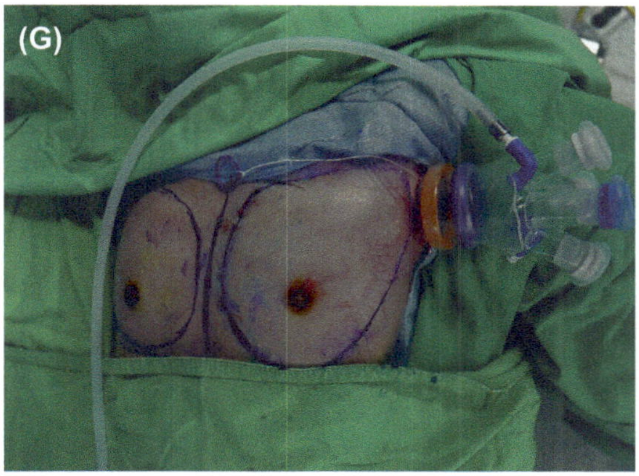

8.19G

Single port insufflation system with CO_2 insufflation to 8 mmHg.

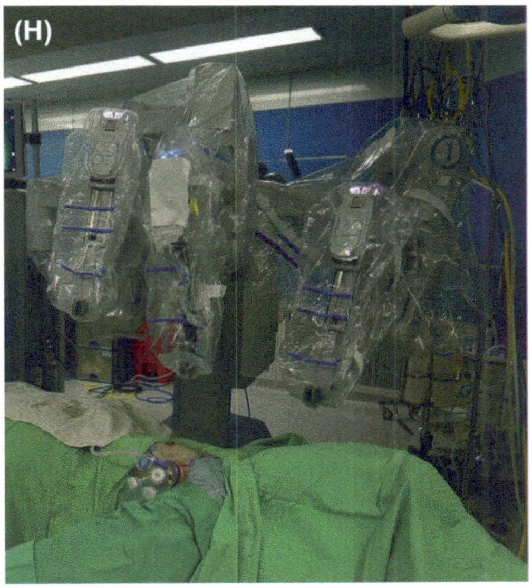

8.19H

Robotic side cart (da Vinci; Intuitive Surgical, Sunnyvale, CA, USA) positioned from the contralateral side, with the robotic arms extending over the patient near the ports before the ports were docked to the arms.

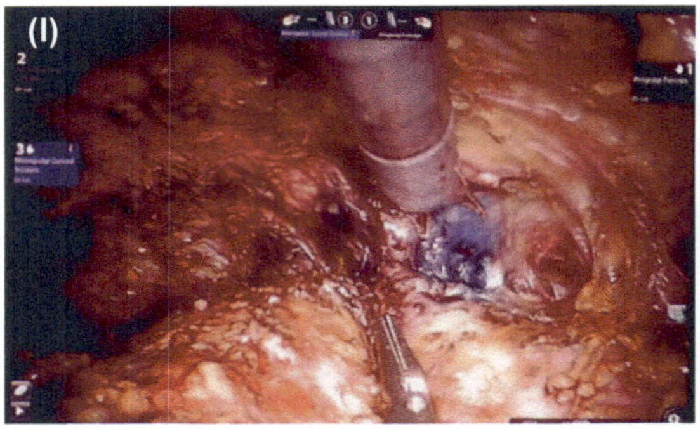

8.19I

3D-view on robotic surgeon console showing dissection of skin flap.

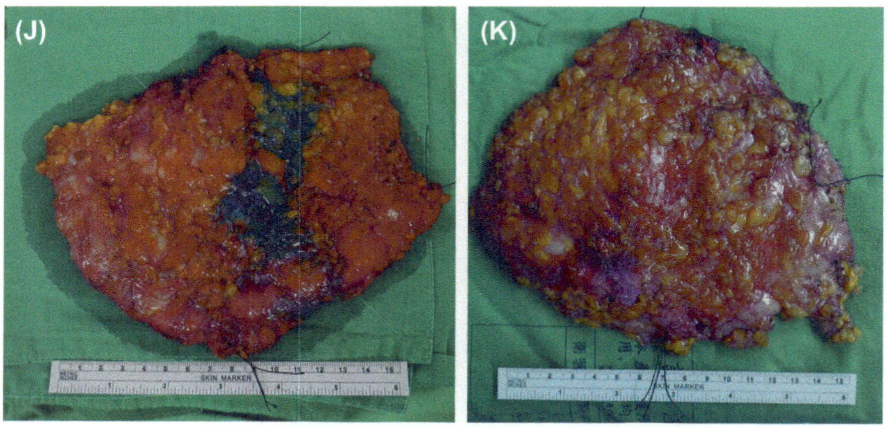

8.19J, K

Mastectomy specimens removed intact and oriented with silk sutures.

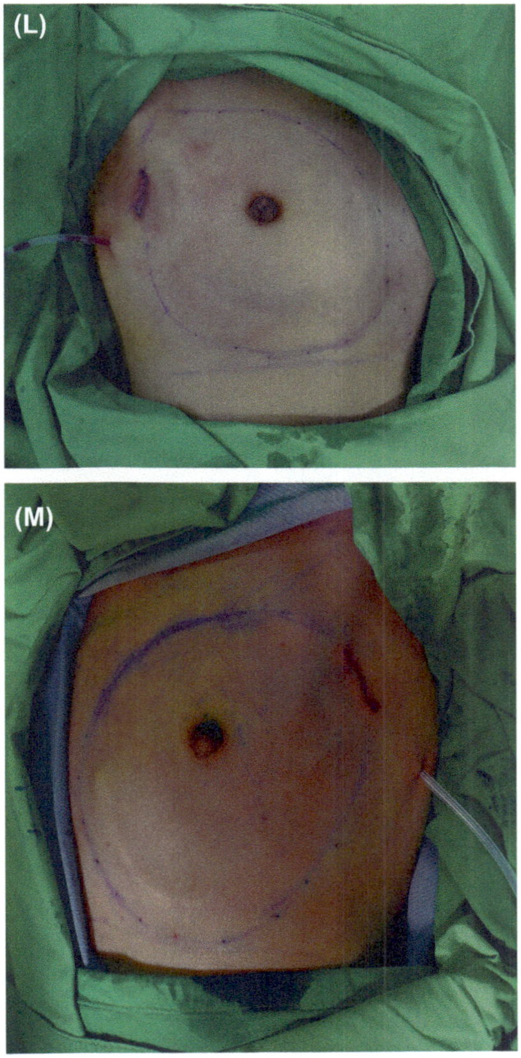

8.19L, M

Immediate post-operative on-table views showing incisions in the axillary region.

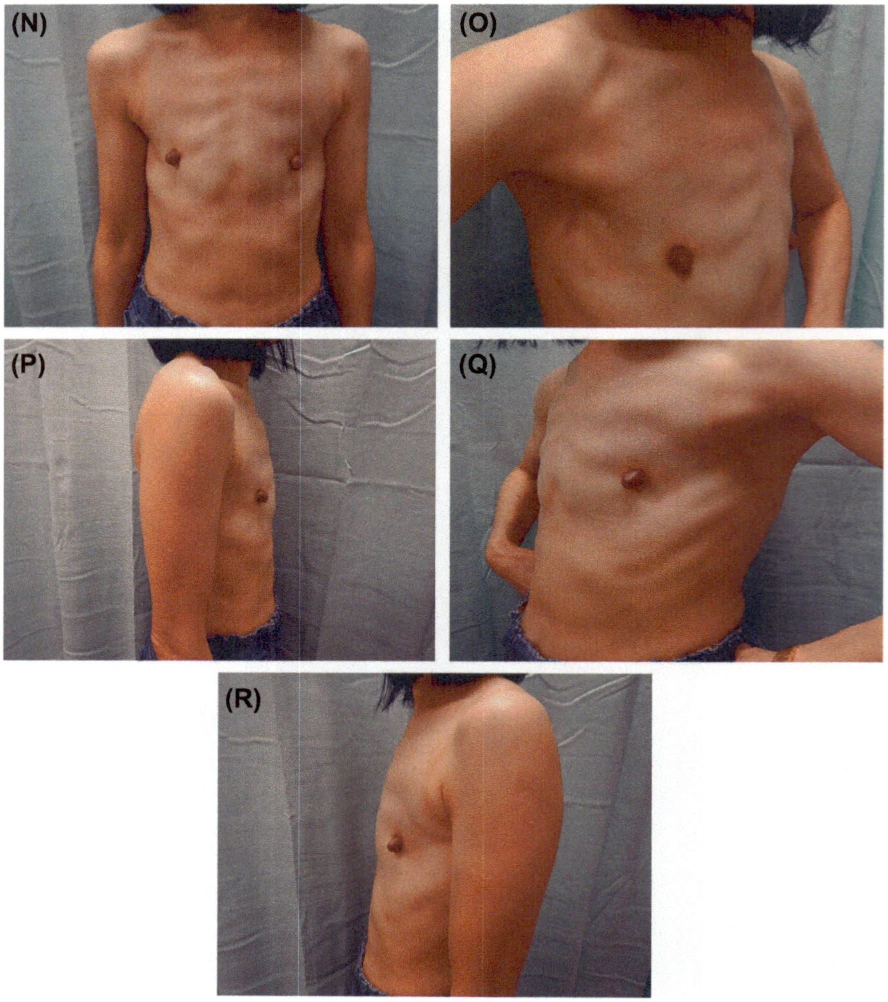

8.19N–R

9 months post-operative views showing well-healed and well-hidden incisions with excellent cosmesis.

Discussion

Robotic surgery, which incorporated three-dimensional imaging system and flexibility of robotic arm and instruments, has seen increasing use in different fields of surgery. R-NSM for therapeutic indications in breast cancer was first reported in 2017 (Toesca et al., 2017). In addition, its use in prophylactic mastectomy was also reported subsequently in a 2018 study (Sarfati et al., 2018). This technique introduces da Vinci surgical platform through a small axillary wound to perform NSM with (or without) immediate breast reconstruction (IBR) and was found to have the potential to overcome the technical difficulty of endoscopic-assisted nipple-sparing mastectomy (E-NSM) and showed promising cosmetic outcome in the authors' experience (Lai, 2019). The inclusion criteria for R-NSM include early-stage breast cancer, tumour size less than 5 cm, no evidence of multiple lymph node metastases, and no evidence of nipple, skin, or chest wall invasion. Patients for whom R-NSM is contraindicated include those with NAC involvement, inflammatory breast cancer, breast cancer with chest wall or skin invasion, locally advanced breast cancer, breast cancer with extensive axillary lymph node metastasis, and patients with severe co-morbid conditions such as heart disease, renal failure, liver dysfunction, and poor performance status as assessed by the primary physicians. Women with large (breast cup size larger than E or breast mastectomy weight >600 g) and ptosis breast are not good candidates for R-NSM and IBR with Gel implant due to technical difficulty and sub-optimal cosmetic outcome. In addition, one of the most common drawbacks in most centres would be cost-related issues, as robotic procedures are still fairly costly compared to other surgical modalities.

References

Lai, H. W. (2019). Robotic nipple-sparing mastectomy and immediate breast reconstruction with Gel implant. *Annals of Surgical Oncology*. https://doi.org/10.1245/s10434-018-6711-3.

Sarfati, B., Struk, S., Leymarie, N., Honart, J. F., Alkhashnam, H., Tran de Fremicourt, K., et al. (2018). Robotic prophylactic nipple-sparing mastectomy with immediate prosthetic breast reconstruction: A prospective study. *Annals of Surgical Oncology*. https://doi.org/10.1245/s10434-018-6555-x.

Toesca, A., Peradze, N., Manconi, A., Galimberti, V., Intra, M., Colleoni, M., et al. (2017). Robotic nipple-sparing mastectomy for the treatment of breast cancer: Feasibility and safety study. *Breast*. https://doi.org/10.1016/j.breast.2016.10.009.

SECTION

2

Robotic breast surgery with reconstruction

CHAPTER 9

Robotic breast-conserving surgery with immediate pedicled latissimus dorsi flap reconstruction

Description of technique

Pre-operative marking and positioning

Pre-operative marking was done with the patient in standing and supine position. After induction of general anaesthesia, the patient was then placed in the supine position and ipsilateral arm abducted to 90 degrees to avoid affecting the operative procedure.

Axillary staging procedure

In patients for whom sentinel lymph node biopsy (SLNB) is indicated, a small amount (2–3 mCi) of radioisotope Tc99m was injected intradermally at the site of the tumour before operation (either on the day or 1 day prior).

After induction of general anaesthesia, 3 mL of 1% methylene blue (Merck, Darmstadt, Germany) was injected into the breast parenchyma in equally divided aliquots at five positions surrounding the hemisphere of the tumour facing the ipsilateral axilla. The breast tissue from the tumour to the axilla was then gently massaged for 5–10 minutes. Within 20–30 minutes after injection of the blue dye, a handheld gamma probe (Navigator; USSC, Norwalk, CT) was used to identify the hot spots and the location of the hottest nodes was then marked. An approximately 3–5 cm oblique axillary incision was then made close to the hottest nodes, and SLNB was then performed. Fresh frozen section was performed as indicated. If SLN was positive for metastases, a complete axillary lymph node dissection up to level II was performed.

Robotic docking, dissection and wide local excision

To create working space for placement of the single port (Glove Port; Nelis Corporation, Gyeonggi-do, Korea), a 3–4 cm subcutaneous flap was dissected with electro cautery under direct vision. The tunnelling technique as described in endoscopic

Minimally Invasive (Endoscopic & Robotic) Breast Surgery. https://doi.org/10.1016/B978-0-323-73405-9.00009-1

mastectomy was then used to facilitate skin flap dissection and create space between the skin flap and the breast parenchyma. Once adequate dissection was achieved, the single port was then inserted through the axilla incision and carbon dioxide (CO_2) insufflation with air pressure kept at 8 mmHg was used to create space for mastectomy. The ipsilateral shoulder was elevated to 30 degrees to prevent conflict between the operating table and docking of the robotic surgery system. The robotic side cart (da Vinci; Intuitive Surgical, Sunnyvale, CA, USA) was then positioned from the contralateral side, with the two robotic arms endoscope extending over the patient near the ports before the ports were docked to the robotic arms. Subsequently, the operation was then shifted to the da Vinci Si or Xi (Intuitive Surgical, Sunnyvale, CA, USA) robotic platform controlled by the operating surgeon at the console. The authors used a 30 degree 12-mm diameter camera (Intuitive Surgical, Denzlingen, Germany) in the upper port to prevent collisions with other instruments. Dissection was carried out using an 8-mm monopolar scissors (Intuitive Surgical, Sunnyvale, CA, USA). Traction and counter-traction, along with maintaining exposure, were carried out using an 8-mm ProGrasp forceps (Intuitive Surgical, Sunnyvale, CA, USA). The location of the scissors and the ProGrasp forceps could be changed inter-variably during the operation. Dissection was initiated from the superficial skin flaps by dissecting the septa between the skin flap and parenchyma created by the tunnelling technique with monopolar scissors. After completion of the superficial skin flap dissection, dissection of the peripheral portion of the breast parenchyma was carried out subsequently. Posterior dissection was then performed by detaching the breast tissue from the pectoralis major muscle fascia with the perforator vessels clearly identified and secured. After development of adequate skin flap, wide excision was completed. To guide resection with adequate margins, the authors recommended the use of intra-operative ultrasound and marking of resection margin with blue dye injection. Specimen was retrieved thereafter and haemostasis secured.

Immediate pedicled latissimus dorsi flap reconstruction

Following removal of the specimen and adequate haemostasis, copious irrigation of the wide excision cavity was performed. Subsequently, the thoracodorsal pedicle was identified and marked with a vessel loop to prevent injury during the flap harvest. The patient was then shifted to the lateral decubitus position. Two 12 mm balloon trocars (Kii Balloon blunt tip system, Applied Medical, Rancho Santa Margarita, CA, USA) were used as working ports. The ports were then docked to the robotic arms, and CO_2 insufflation was applied at 10–12 mmHg. Dissection was started along the under surface of the latissimus dorsi (LD) muscle. Blood vessels encountered were carefully dissected, coagulated and cut with monopolar scissors. As the dissection through the under surface of the muscle to the borders was completed, further dissection over the superficial surface of the muscle ensued.

The muscle was disconnected from the infero-posterior and scapular border. Afterwards, the pedicled LD flap was exteriorized from the axilla wound and the robotic arms were then undocked. Reconstruction of the wide excision defect was performed with the patient turned back to a supine position. Fixation of the flap to the breast parenchyma was performed with assistance from a handle light retractor to ensure full coverage of the defect. Care must be taken to ensure the correct axis of the vascular pedicle to prevent torsion of the blood supply. Drains were then placed both in the donor site and in the wide excision cavity.

Case 20: robotic breast-conserving surgery with immediate pedicled latissimus dorsi flap reconstruction – single axillary incision

Patient/demographics

This case described a 28-year-old female who presented with a palpable mass over her left breast. Sonography revealed a suspicious mass about 6 cm in which core needle biopsies performed subsequently showed a triple negative breast cancer (TNBC). Breast magnetic resonance imaging (MRI) was performed, and no other suspicious lesions were seen. Her metastatic workup was negative. In view of TNBC and the size of primary tumor, patient underwent neoadjuvant chemotherapy uneventfully with partial response on subsequent breast MRI. During pre-operative consultation, the patient expressed a strong desire for breast conservation. Left upper outer quadrantectomy was suggested with immediate pedicled latissimus dorsi (LD) flap reconstruction.

Surgery and pathology report

The patient subsequently underwent robotic-assisted breast-conserving surgery with sentinel lymph node biopsy with immediate pedicled LD flap reconstruction. Sentinel lymph node biopsy for the frozen section was negative. The final pathology reported invasive ductal carcinoma with medullary features, ypT2N0M0 (stage IIA) with clear margins. She received adjuvant radiotherapy.

Post-operative outcomes

Post-operation recovery was uneventful except for seroma formation over the donor site, which was relieved after repeated aspiration in outpatient setting. The patient was satisfied with the post-operative scar and aesthetic outcome.

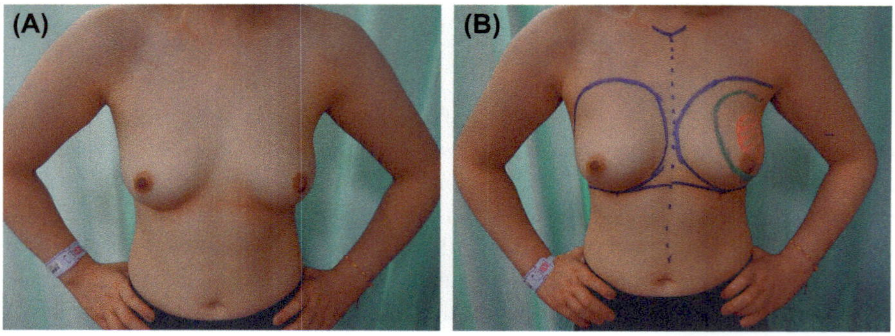

9.20A, B

Pre-operative front views showing pre-operative markings and tumor location.

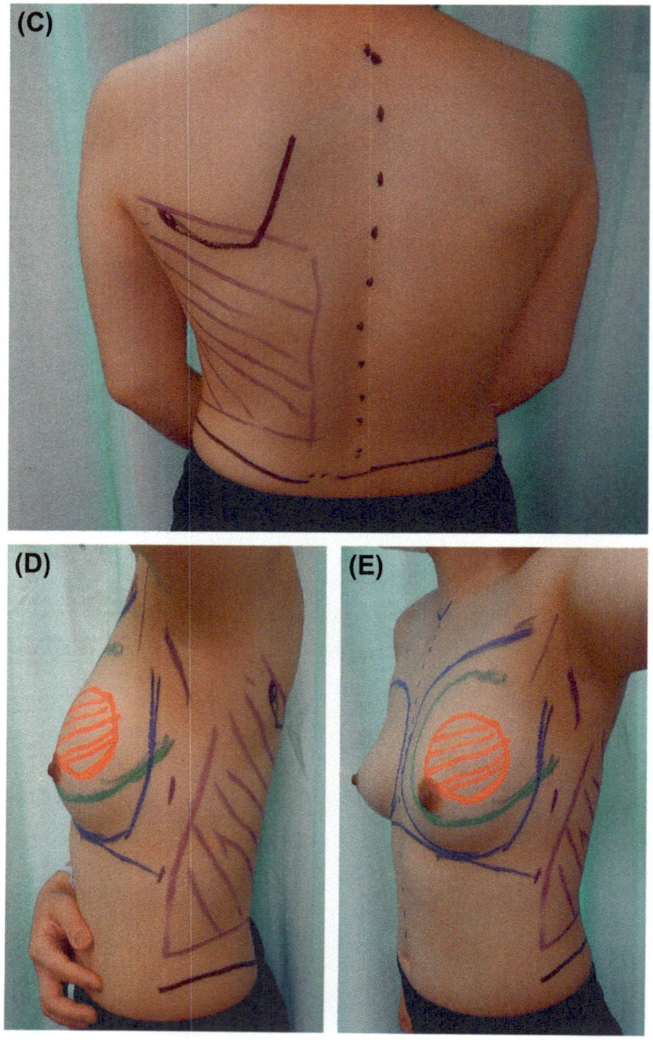

9.20C–E

Pre-operative markings showing planned dissection for LD flap and incisions.

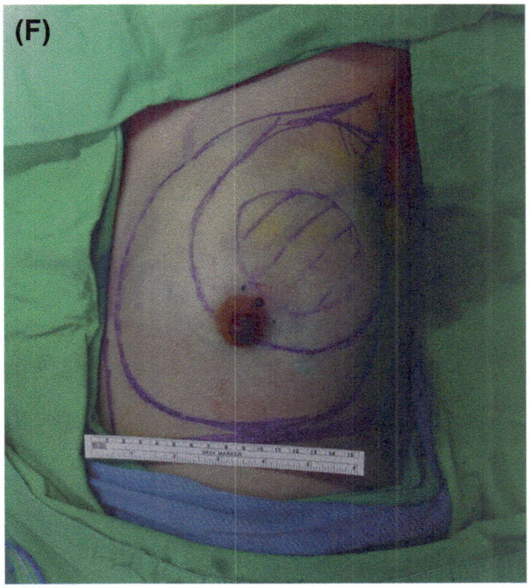

9.20F

On-table view showing planned resection margins for quadrantectomy.

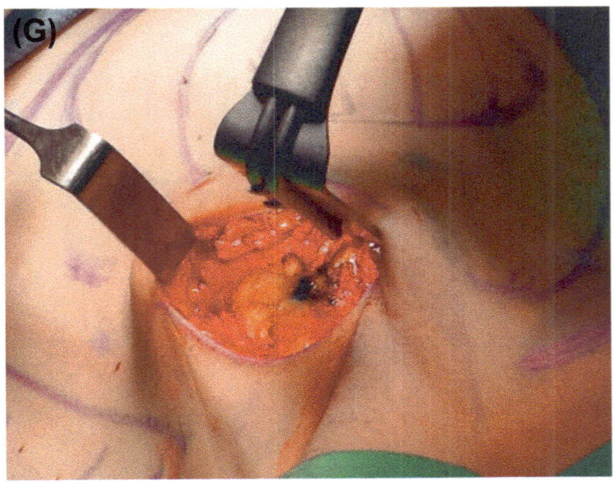

9.20G

Sentinel lymph node biopsy performed via axillary incision.

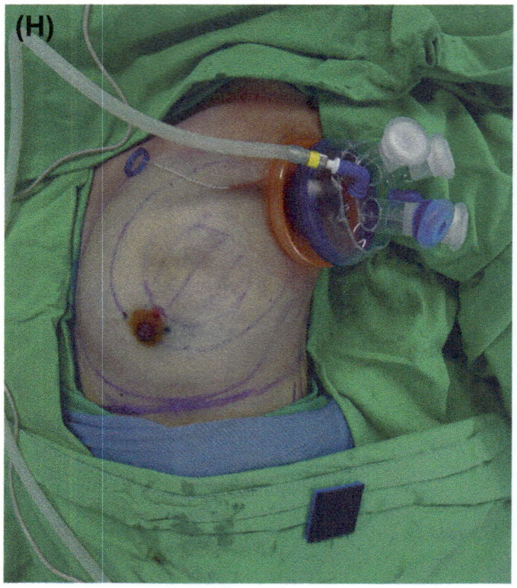

9.20H

After creation of the working space, a single port (Glove Port, Nelis, Gyeonggi-do, Korea) was placed with CO_2 insufflation to 8 mmHg.

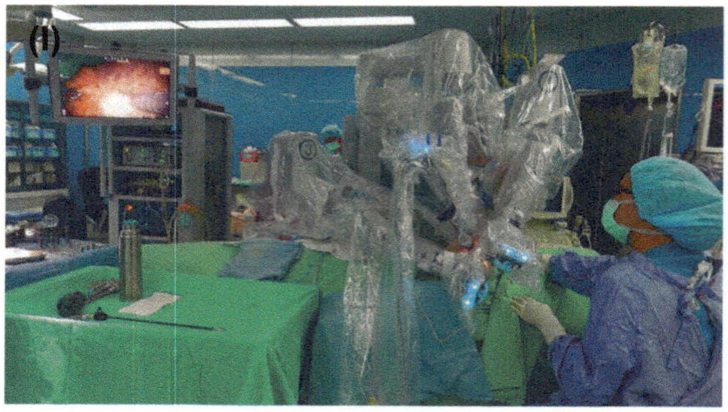

9.20I

Operating theater view showing the intra-operative setting, which was performed with a da Vinci Si (Intuitive Surgical, Sunnyvale, CA) robotic platform with the operating surgeon controlling at the surgeon's console.

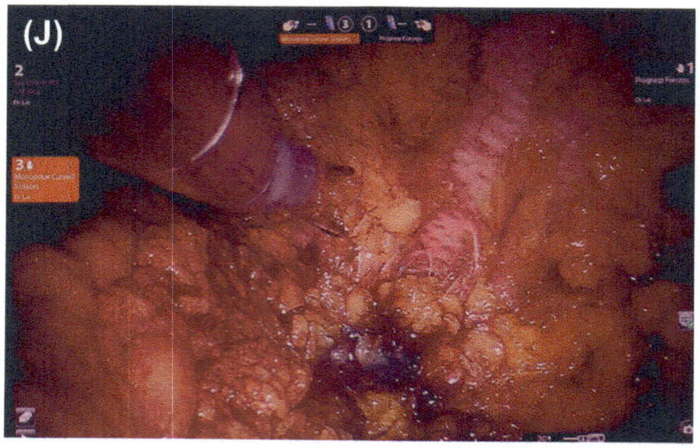

9.20J

Anterior skin flap dissection was performed by dissecting septa off the skin and breast parenchyma with monopolar scissors.

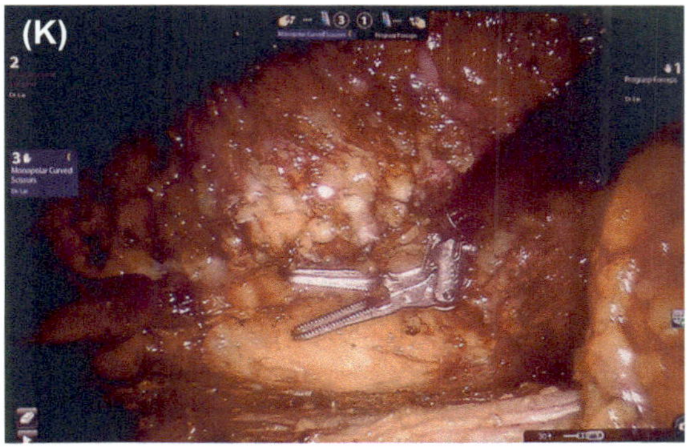

9.20K

After peripheral dissection and parenchyma resection, left upper outer quadrantectomy was completed.

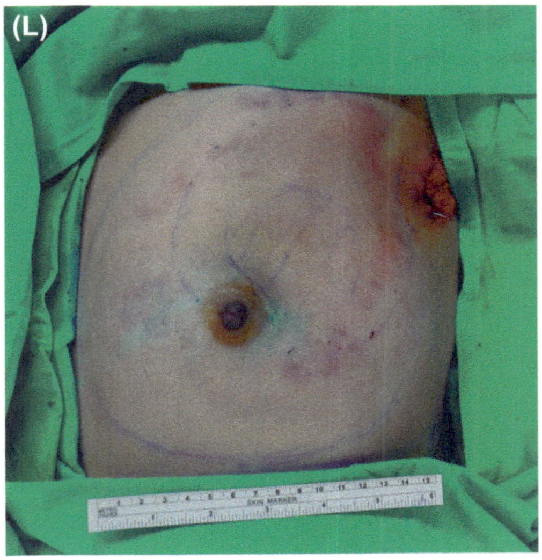

9.20L

Immediate on-table view after quadrantectomy.

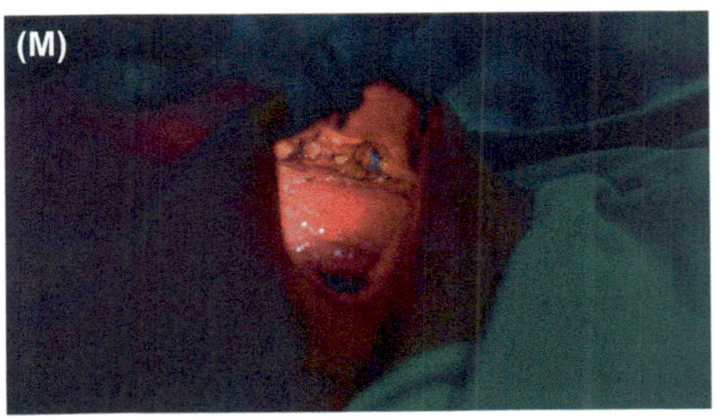

9.20M

Direct view of resection cavity seen.

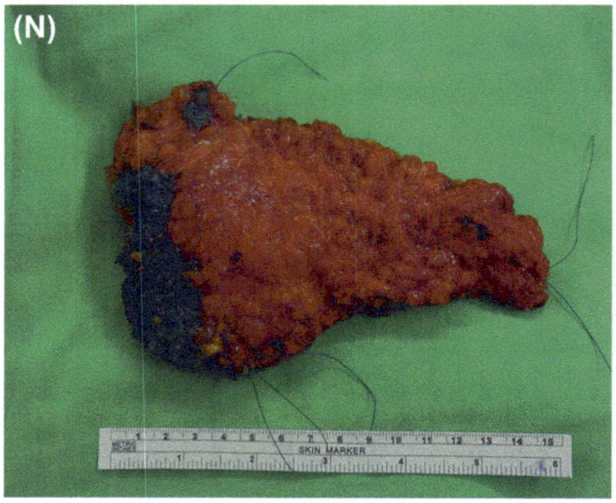

9.20N

The entire resected quadrantectomy breast specimen intact and oriented.

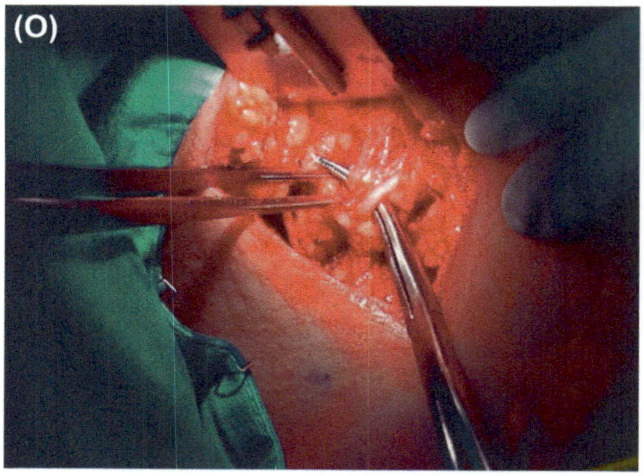

9.20O

Thoracodorsal bundle identified via axillary incision and marked with a vessel loop.

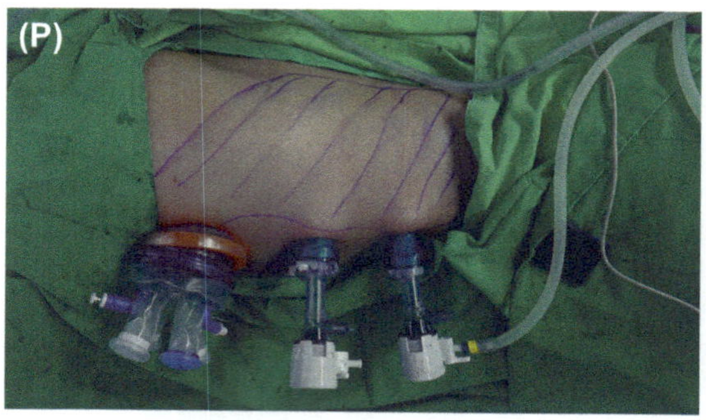

9.20P

Patient was then shifted to lateral decubitus position with two more working ports placed along the mid-axillary line.

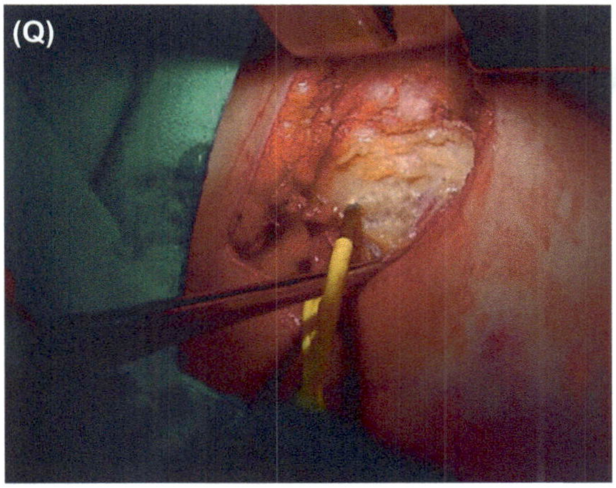

9.20Q

Dissection of the flap started from the undersurface of the muscle.

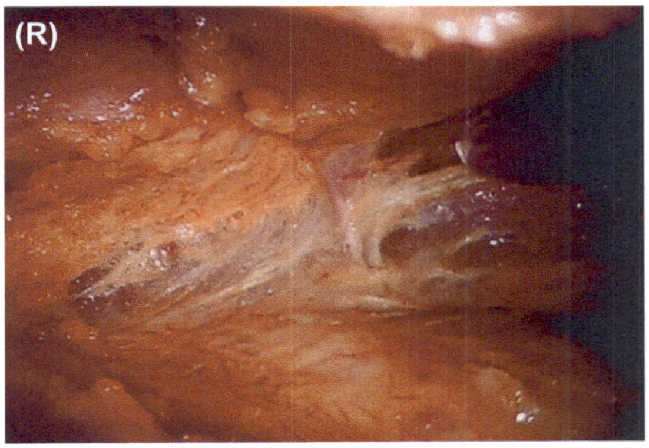

9.20R

After the undersurface of the muscle was dissected to the borders, dissection was then advanced over the superficial surface of the muscle.

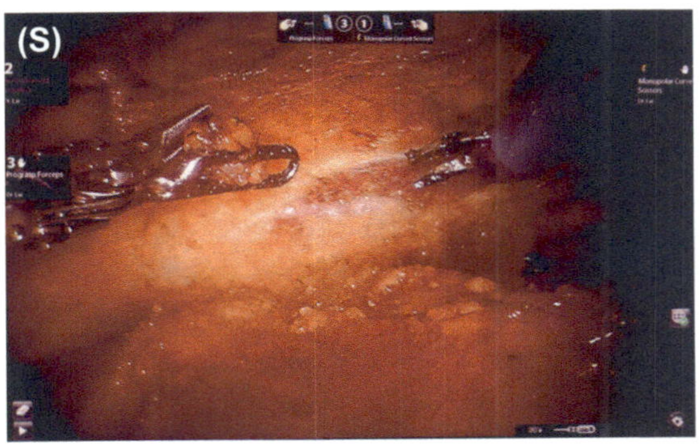

9.20S

Once dissection is complete along both the deep and superficial surfaces, monopolar scissors are used to disinsert the muscle from the inferoposterior border.

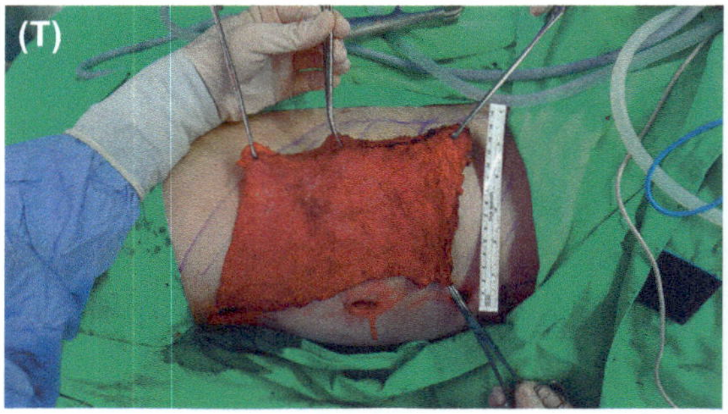

9.20T

The pedicled latissimus dorsi flap, which was harvested by robotic means, was ready for transfer to post mastectomy subcutaneous space.

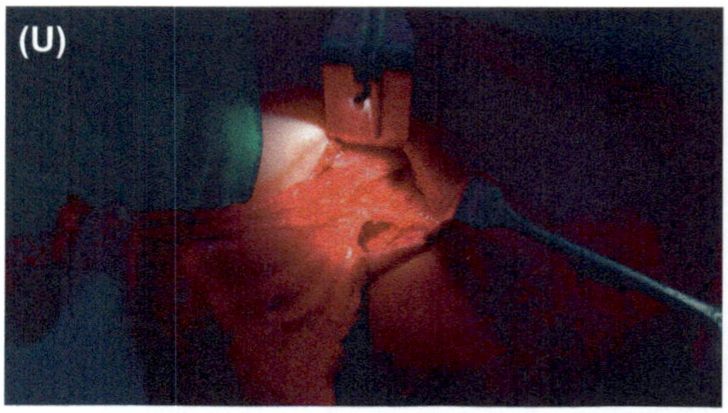

9.20U

Pedicle well protected as shown here.

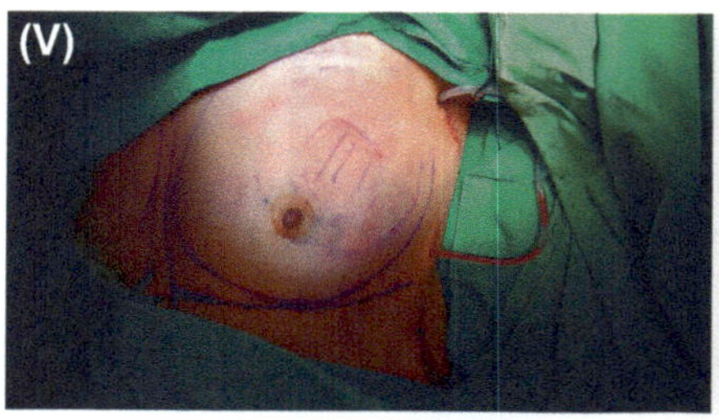

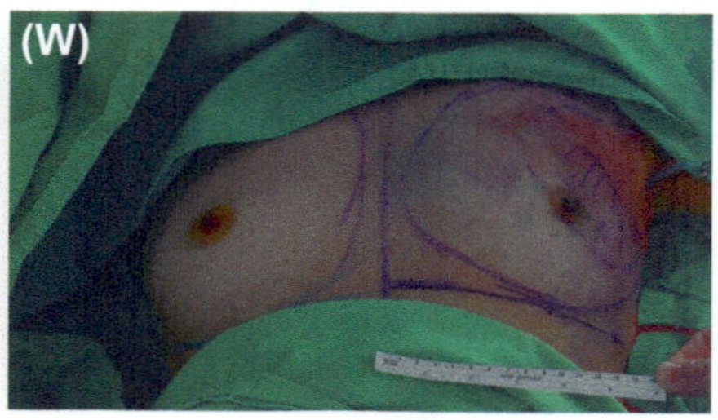

9.20V, W

Immediate on-table post-operative views showing small, inconspicuous wounds.

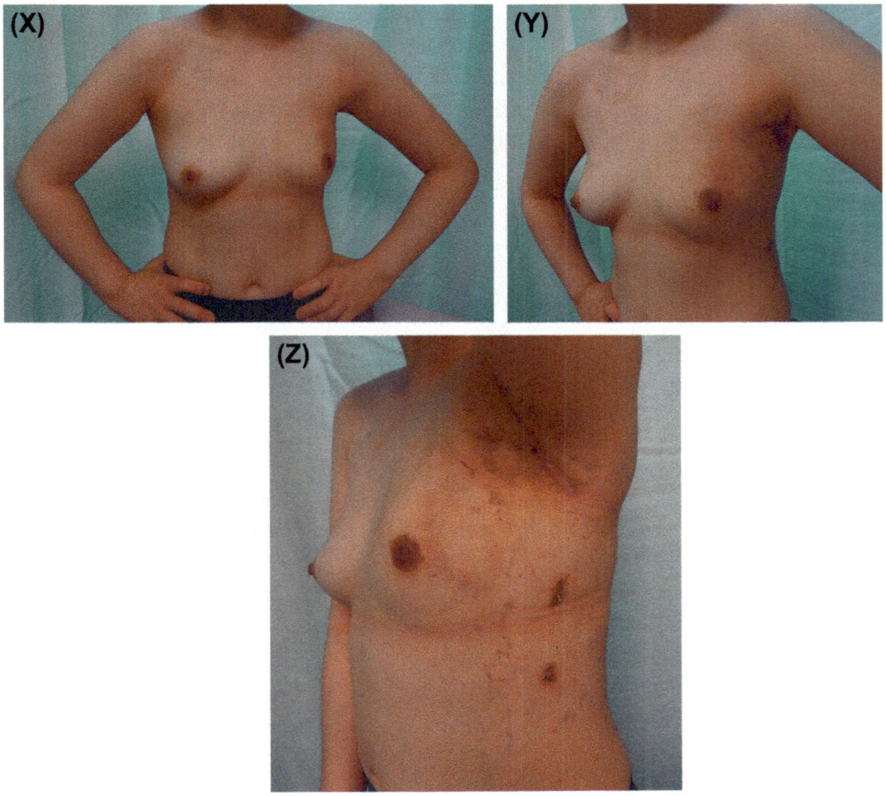

9.20X–Z

1-month post-operative views showing well-healed scars and satisfactory cosmesis and symmetry.

Discussion

Pedicled LD flap has been widely used in breast reconstruction procedures (Sood, Easow, Konopka, & Panthaki, 2018). A long scar on the back, which is usually 15–25 cm in length, can be avoided by endoscopic or robotic-assisted LD flap harvest in cases whereby skin island is not needed as part of the reconstruction. Robotic-assisted harvest, which was first reported in 2012 (Selber, Baumann, & Holsinger, 2012) has gradually replaced endoscopic-assisted method because it overcomes some of the limitations and technical difficulties of endoscopic harvesting. In the authors' experience (Lai et al., 2018), robotic-assisted harvesting has the advantage of three-dimensional vision, flexibility of instruments of the da Vinci operating system. The technique is suitable for early breast cancer patients with small to medium-sized breast who desire breast conservation. LD flap is one of the most reliable flaps for volume replacement and is often indicated when the resected volume is greater than 150 g. The post-operative cosmetic result is good with the avoidance of a long donor site scar. The most frequently encountered complications of conventional LD flap harvest will be seroma formation and wound-related complications which is greatly reduced in robotic-assisted LD flap harvest.

References

Lai, H. W., Chen, S. T., Lin, S. L., Lin, Y. L., Wu, H. K., Pai, S. H., et al. (2018). Technique for single axillary incision robotic assisted quadrantectomy and immediate partial breast reconstruction with robotic latissimus dorsi flap harvest for breast cancer. *Medicine (United States)*. https://doi.org/10.1097/MD.0000000000011373.

Selber, J. C., Baumann, D. P., & Holsinger, F. C. (2012). Robotic latissimus dorsi muscle harvest: A case series. *Plastic and Reconstructive Surgery*. https://doi.org/10.1097/PRS.0b013e31824ecc0b.

Sood, R., Easow, J. M., Konopka, G., & Panthaki, Z. J. (2018). Latissimus dorsi flap in breast reconstruction: Recent innovations in the workhorse flap. *Cancer Control*. https://doi.org/10.1177/1073274817744638.

CHAPTER

Robotic mastectomy with immediate implant reconstruction

10

Description of technique

Pre-operative marking and positioning

Pre-operative marking was done with the patient in standing and supine position. After induction of general anaesthesia, the patient was then placed in the supine position and ipsilateral arm abducted to 90 degrees to avoid affecting the operative procedure.

Axillary staging procedure

In patients for whom sentinel lymph node biopsy (SLNB) is indicated, a small amount (2−3 mCi) of radioisotope Tc99m was injected intradermally at the site of the tumour before operation (either on the day or 1 day prior).

After induction of general anaesthesia, 3 mL of 1% methylene blue (Merck, Darmstadt, Germany) was injected into the breast parenchyma in equally divided aliquots at five positions surrounding the hemisphere of the tumour facing the ipsilateral axilla. The breast tissue from the tumour to the axilla was then gently massaged for 5−10 minutes. Within 20−30 minutes after injection of the blue dye, a handheld gamma probe (Navigator; USSC, Norwalk, CT) was used to identify the hot spots and the location of the hottest nodes was then marked. An approximately 3−5 cm oblique axillary incision was then made close to the hottest nodes, and SLNB was then performed. Fresh frozen section was performed as indicated. If SLN was positive for metastases, a complete axillary lymph node dissection up to level II was performed.

Robotic docking and dissection

To create working space for placement of the single port (Glove Port; Nelis Corporation, Gyeonggi-do, Korea), a 3−4 cm subcutaneous flap was dissected with electrocautery under direct vision. The tunnelling technique as described in endoscopic mastectomy was then used to facilitate skin flap dissection and create space between the skin flap and the breast parenchyma. Once adequate dissection was achieved, the

Minimally Invasive (Endoscopic & Robotic) Breast Surgery. https://doi.org/10.1016/B978-0-323-73405-9.00010-8

single port was then inserted through the axilla incision, and carbon dioxide (CO_2) insufflation with air pressure kept at 8 mmHg was used to create space for mastectomy. The ipsilateral shoulder was elevated to 30 degrees to prevent conflict between the operating table and docking of the robotic surgery system. The robotic side cart (da Vinci; Intuitive Surgical, Sunnyvale, CA, USA) was then positioned from the contralateral side, with the two robotic arms endoscope extending over the patient near the ports before the ports were docked to the robotic arms. Subsequently, the operation was then shifted to the da Vinci Si or Xi (Intuitive Surgical, Sunnyvale, CA, USA) robotic platform controlled by the operating surgeon at the console. The authors used a 30 degree 12-mm diameter camera (Intuitive Surgical, Denzlingen, Germany) in the upper port to prevent collisions with other instruments. Dissection was carried out using an 8-mm monopolar scissors (Intuitive Surgical, Sunnyvale, CA, USA). Traction and counter-traction, along with maintaining exposure, were carried out using an 8-mm ProGrasp forceps (Intuitive Surgical, Sunnyvale, CA, USA). The location of the scissors and the ProGrasp forceps could be changed inter-variably during the operation. Dissection was initiated from the superficial skin flaps by dissecting the septa between the skin flap and parenchyma created by the tunnelling technique with monopolar scissors. A sub-areolar biopsy and fresh frozen section analysis can be performed in a nipple-sparing mastectomy (NSM). If cancer cell invasion was found in the sub-areolar area, the entire nipple-areola complex (NAC) was removed and conversion to a skin-sparing mastectomy was then performed. After completion of the superficial skin flap dissection, dissection of the peripheral portion of the breast parenchyma was carried out subsequently. Posterior dissection was then performed by detaching the breast tissue from the pectoralis major muscle fascia with the perforator vessels clearly identified and secured. After completion of dissection, the entire breast specimen was removed through the axillary wound.

Immediate implant reconstruction

Following removal of the specimen and adequate haemostasis, copious irrigation of the mastectomy pocket was performed. Subsequently, the lateral border of the pectoralis major muscle was elevated to allow for sub-muscular pocket dissection. The working space was developed under direct vision by electrocautery with assistance of a handle light retractor. The single port was then re-inserted with CO_2 insufflation for robotic sub-muscular pocket dissection using a da Vinci surgical platform. Dissection was performed medially towards the sternal border, taking care not to injure the perforator vessels. Inferiorly, the dissection was carried out beyond the inframammary fold over the lateral aspect, below which the muscle was released to continue the dissection to the subcutaneous plane thus allowing for a more natural placement of the implant. In the lateral border, the superficial fascia of the serratus anterior muscle was dissected posteriorly in a limited fashion so that it was just enough to accommodate the lateral border of the implant. After initial dissection of the sub-muscular space with the da Vinci surgical platform, the robotic instruments and single port were removed. The operating table was then moved into the sitting position. The adequacy of the sub-muscular pocket dissection was checked and completed with the assistance of a light source retractor. After creation of the sub-muscular pocket, an implant (Mentor Worldwide LLC, Santa Barbara, CA) was then placed followed by drains placement in both sub-muscular and subcutaneous planes. Care was taken when tagging the free muscle edges laterally.

Case 21: Robotic nipple-sparing mastectomy with immediate implant reconstruction – single incision

Patient/demographics

This is a case of a 53-year-old lady who presented with a hard lump in her left breast. Core biopsy pre-operatively revealed an invasive ductal carcinoma, ER+, PR-, CerbB+

Her metastatic workup was negative.

The patient opted for mastectomy with immediate reconstruction, and she was offered a robotic nipple-sparing mastectomy with implant reconstruction.

Surgery and pathology report

The patient underwent a robotic nipple-sparing mastectomy, sentinel lymph node biopsy, and implant reconstruction. Intra-operative frozen section for sentinel lymph node and sub-nipple biopsies were both negative.

Her final histology reported a stage IIA disease (T2N0M0), and she subsequently received adjuvant chemotherapy and endocrine therapy for 5 years.

Post-operative outcomes

Her post-op recovery was uneventful, and she was satisfied with her post-operative cosmesis.

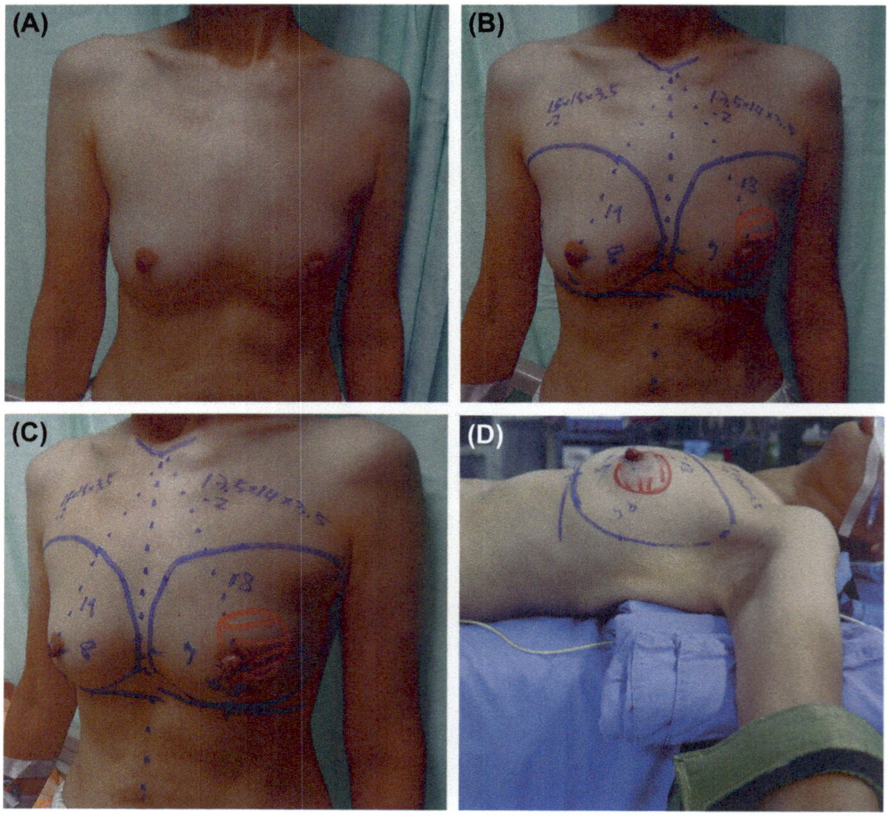

10.21A–D

Pre-operative views showing markings and tumor location as well as positioning of patient.

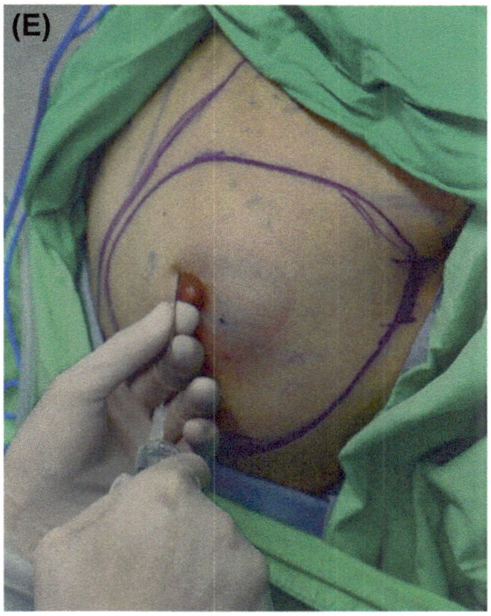

10.21E

A physiological saline solution containing lidocaine 0.05% and epinephrine 1:1,000,000 was injected subcutaneously into the whole breast to minimize bleeding.

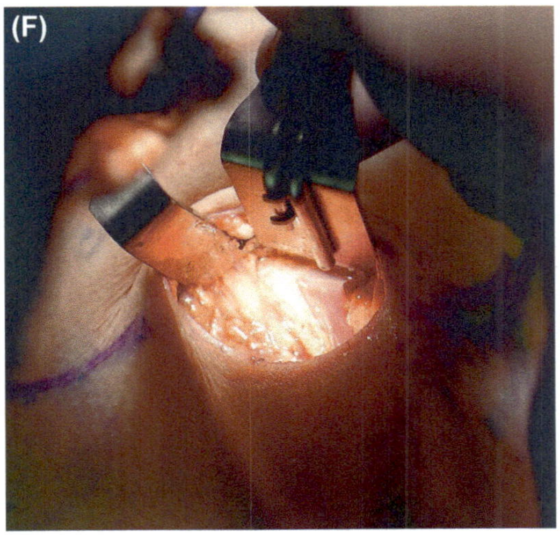

10.21F

Sentinel lymph node biopsy performed via axillary incision.

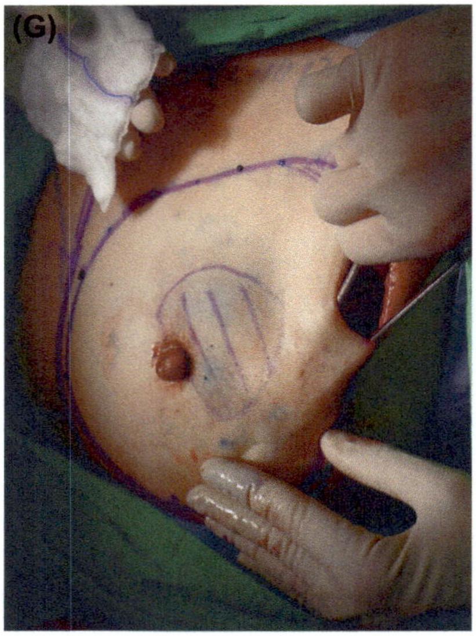

10.21G

Blunt dissection with tissue scissors to aid in plane dissection – tunneling technique.

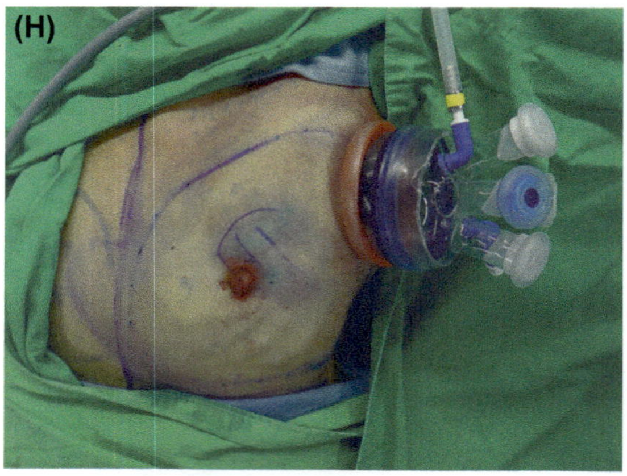

10.21H

After creation of the working space, a single port (Glove Port, Nelis, Gyeonggi-do, Korea) was placed with CO_2 insufflation to 8 mmHg.

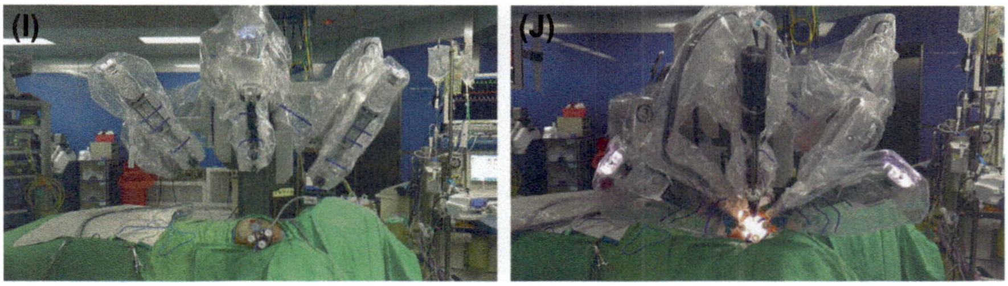

10.21I, J

Operating theater view showing the intra-operative setting, which was performed with a da Vinci Si (Intuitive Surgical, Sunnyvale, CA) robotic platform with the operating surgeon controlling at the surgeon's console.

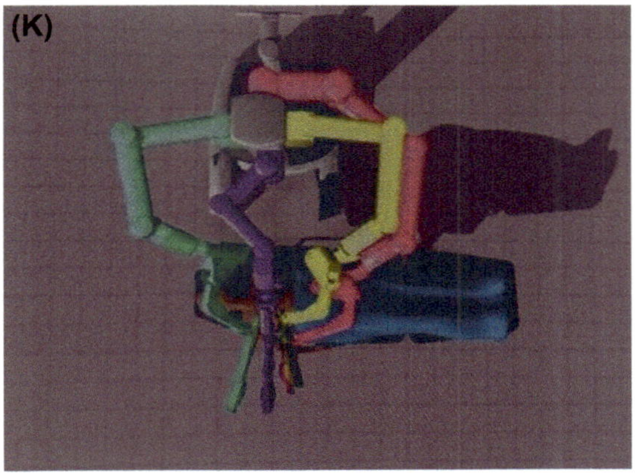

10.21K

To prevent conflicts during dissection the elbows of robotic arms were opened as wide as possible.

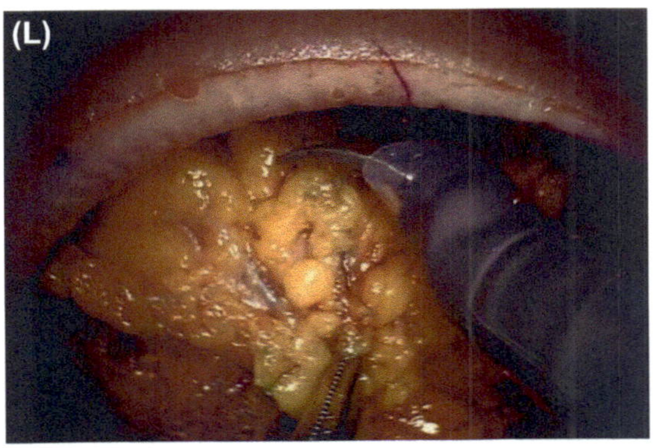

10.21L

Dissection of skin flap with monopolar scissors.

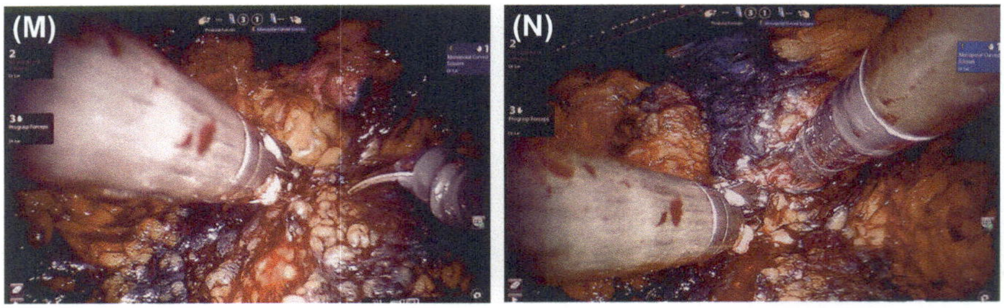

10.21M, N

Intra-operative sub-nipple biopsies performed for the frozen section analysis.

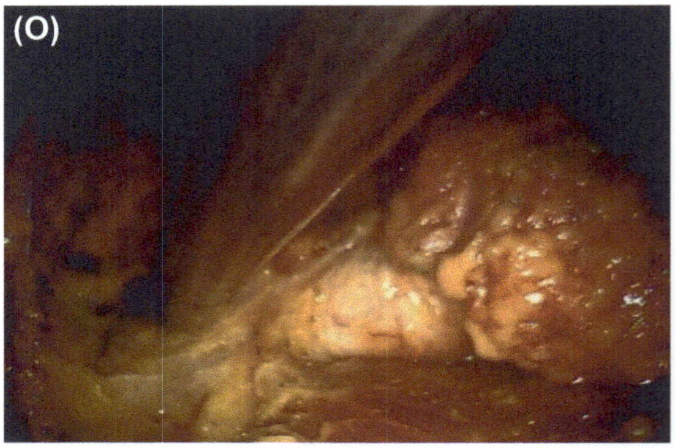

10.21O

After completion of superficial skin flap dissection, the peripheral and posterior dissection was performed.

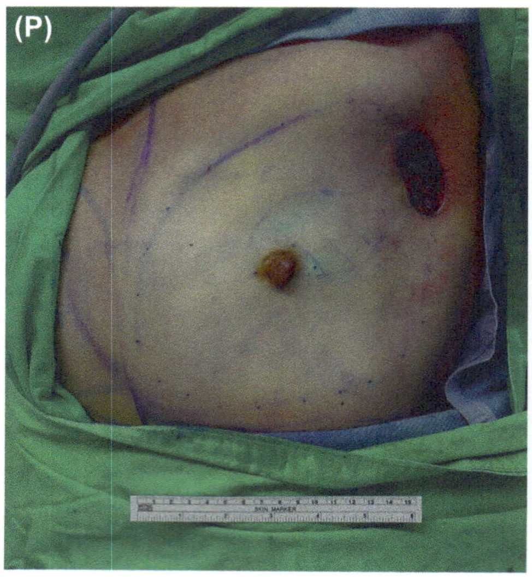

10.21P

Completion of nipple-sparing mastectomy along planned resection margins.

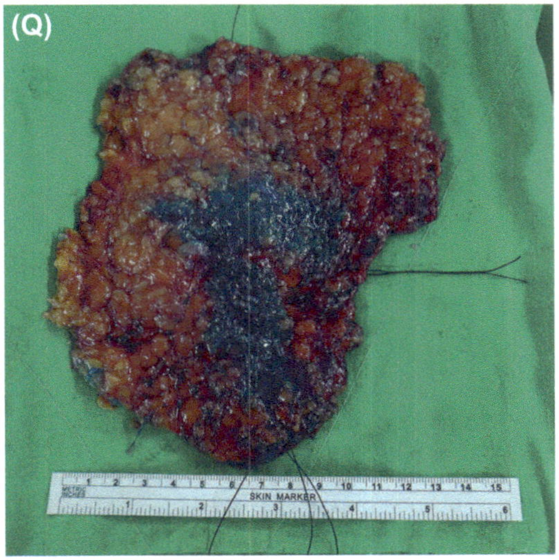

10.21Q

Mastectomy specimen removed intact and oriented.

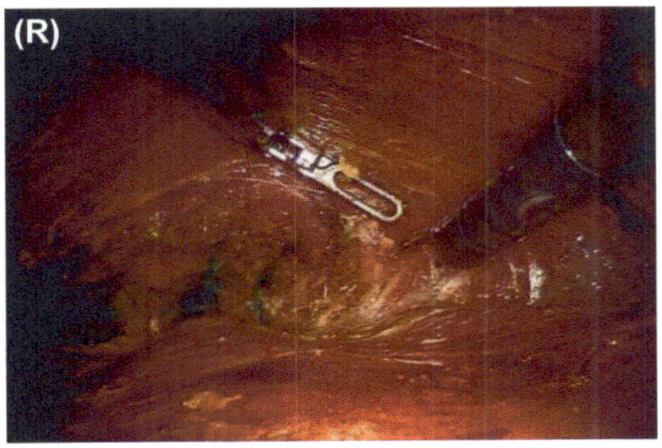

10.21R

Submuscular pocket dissection with prograsp forceps and monopolar scissors.

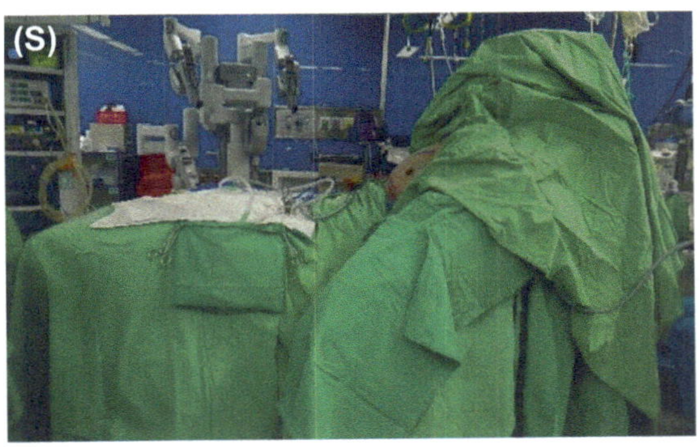

10.21S

Patient was placed in a semi-recumbent position to aid with implant placement.

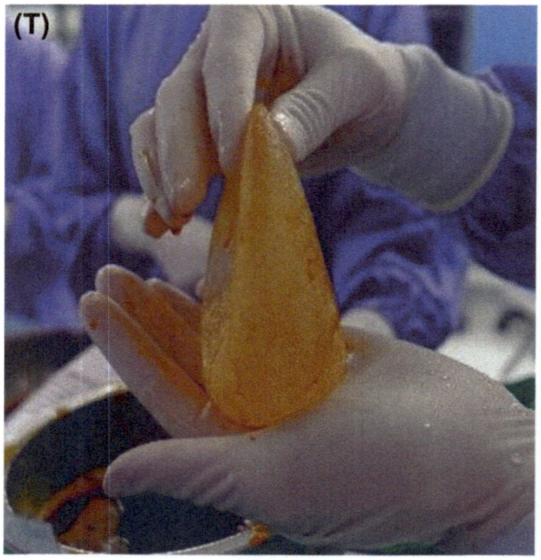

10.21T

Anatomical gel implant for immediate reconstruction.

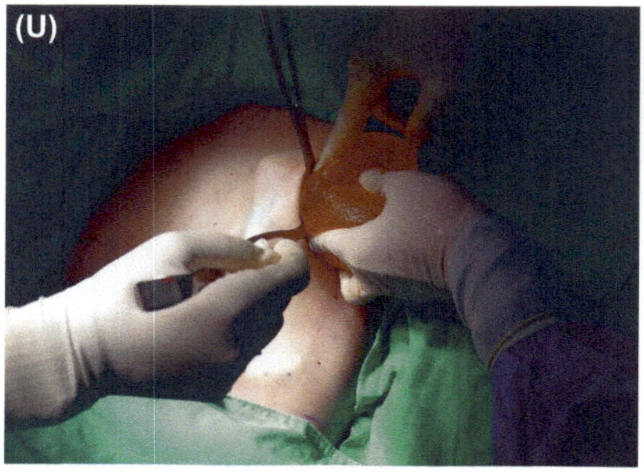

10.21U

Gel implant was inserted from the axillary incision and placed in the submuscular pocket.

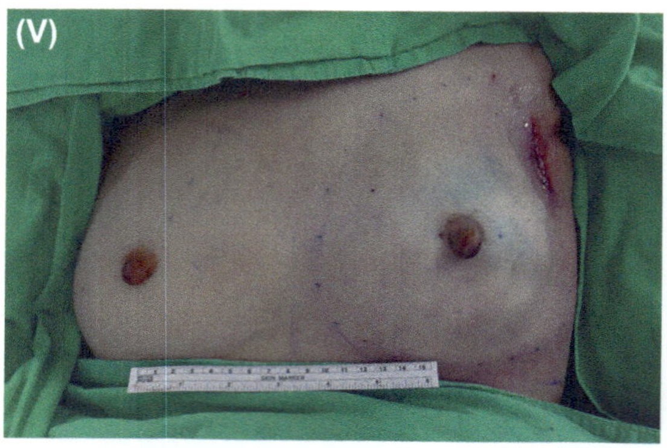

10.21V

Immediate on-table view after implant placement.

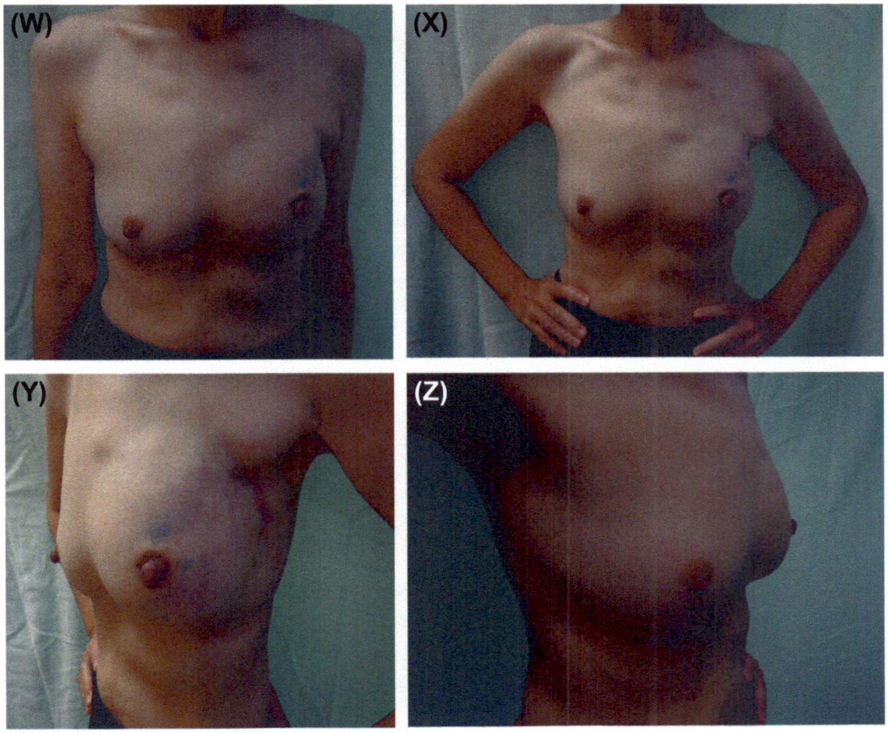

10.21W–Z

2 weeks post-operative views showing well-healed wound and good symmetry.

Case 22: Robotic nipple-sparing mastectomy with immediate implant reconstruction – single incision, previous breast augmentation with silicone implant

Patient/demographics

The case described a 35-year-old lady diagnosed with right breast cancer with a pre-operative core biopsy report of an invasive ductal carcinoma with mucinous features. ER/PR+, CerbB2+.

Her metastatic workup did not reveal any distant metastases.

The patient had bilateral breast augmentation done 5 years before current presentation.

She decided for a robotic nipple-sparing mastectomy with immediate implant reconstruction and counseled for placement of a new implant thereafter.

Surgery and pathology report

The patient underwent right robotic nipple-sparing mastectomy with sentinel lymph node biopsy and immediate implant reconstruction. Intra-operative frozen section for sentinel lymph node and sub-nipple biopsies were negative.

Her final histology reported T2N0M0 (stage IIA) disease, and she received adjuvant chemotherapy and endocrine therapy for 5 years.

Post-operative outcomes

She was discharged 3 days after her operation with an uneventful post-operative recovery thereafter. The patient was reviewed at regular intervals after operation, and her post-operative cosmesis was graded as excellent.

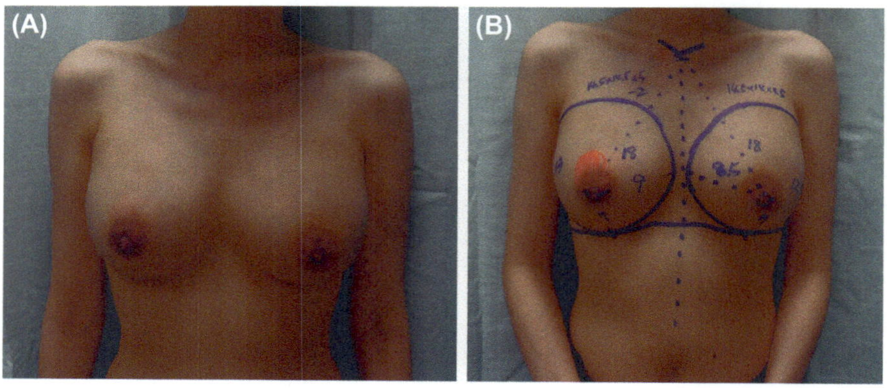

10.22A, B

Pre-operative front views with markings showing tumor location.

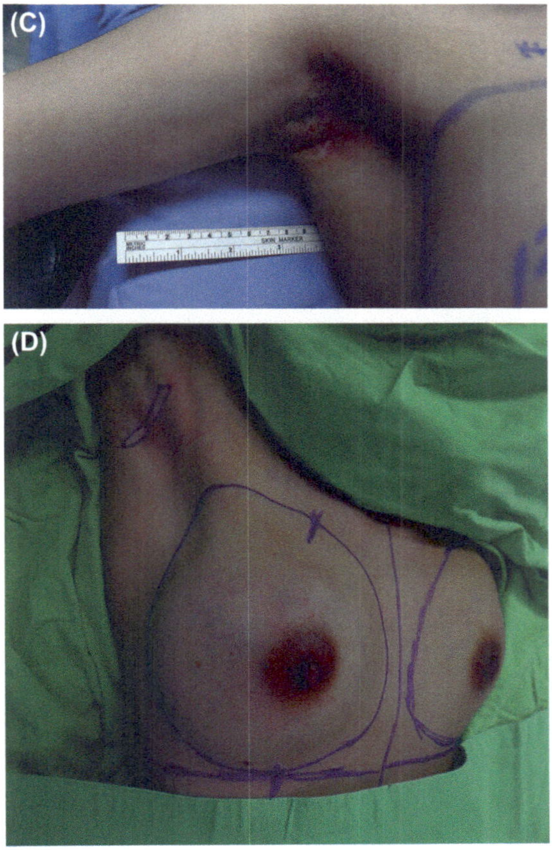

10.22C, D

Previous augmentation scar used as incision for the operation.

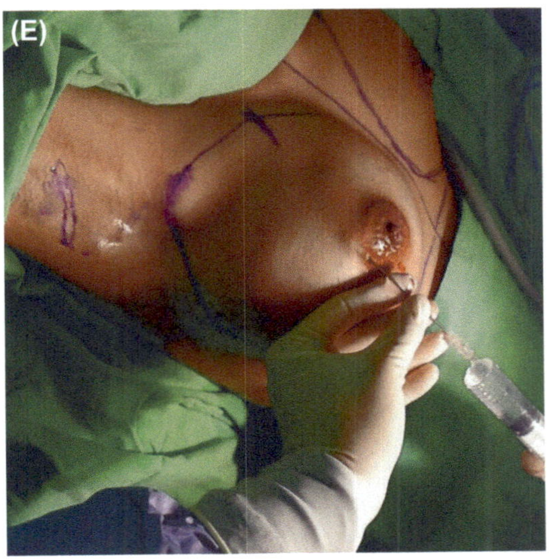

10.22E

A physiological saline solution containing lidocaine 0.05% and epinephrine 1:1,000,000 was injected subcutaneously into the whole breast to minimize bleeding.

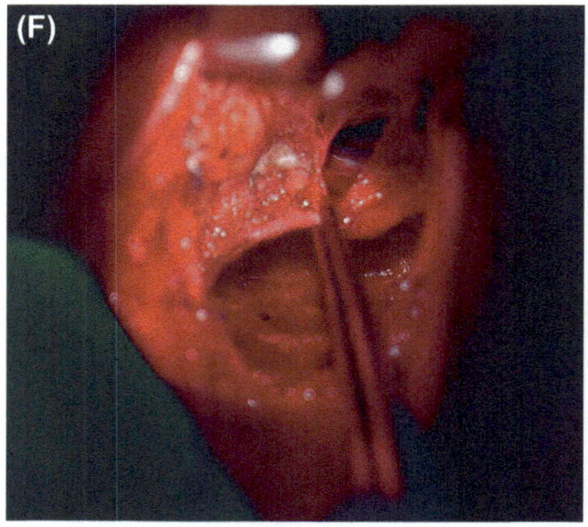

10.22F

Dissection toward the implant after completion of sentinel lymph biopsy.

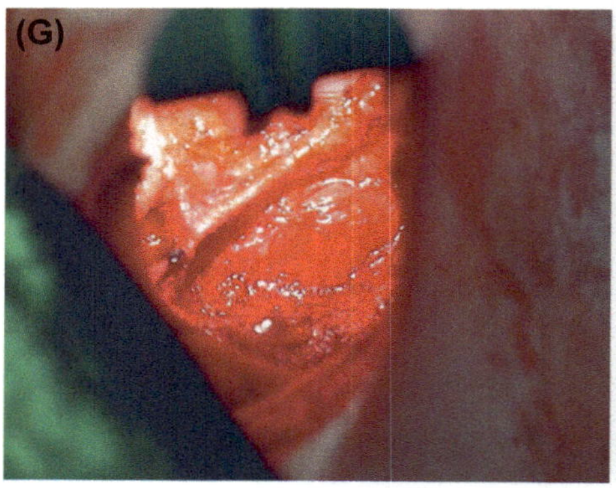

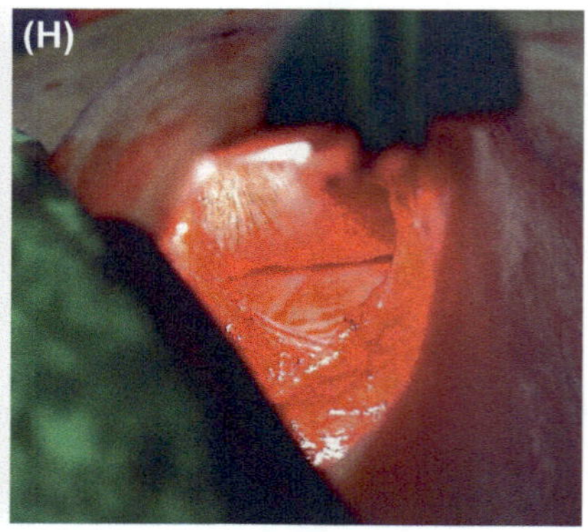

10.22G, H

Submuscular pocket seen after removal of implant.

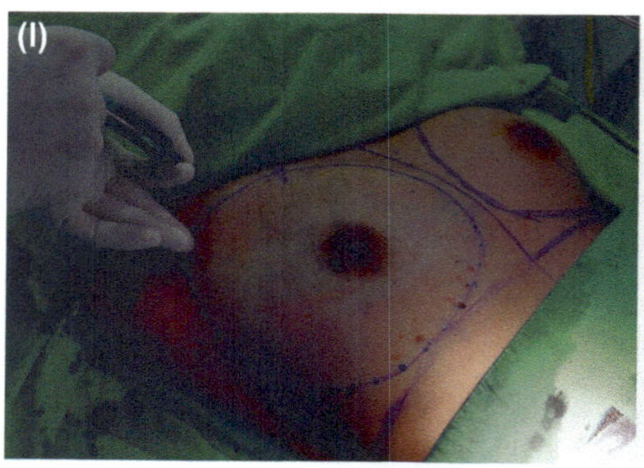

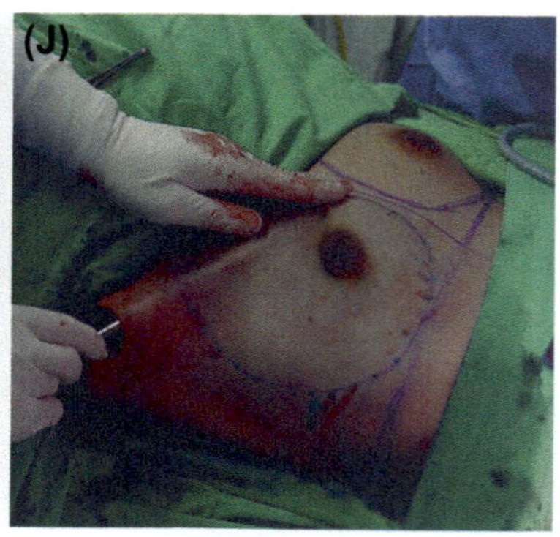

10.22I, J

Blue dye used to mark out dissection margins. Blunt dissection with tissue scissors to aid in plane dissection, also known as tunneling technique.

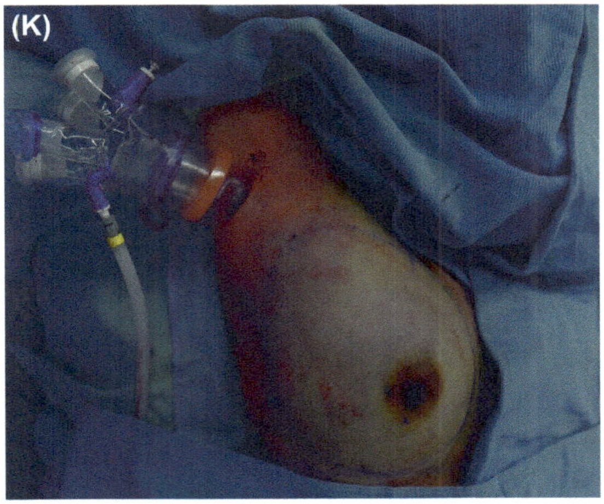

10.22K

After creation of the working space, a single port (Glove Port, Nelis, Gyeonggi-do, Korea) was placed with CO_2 insufflation to 8 mmHg.

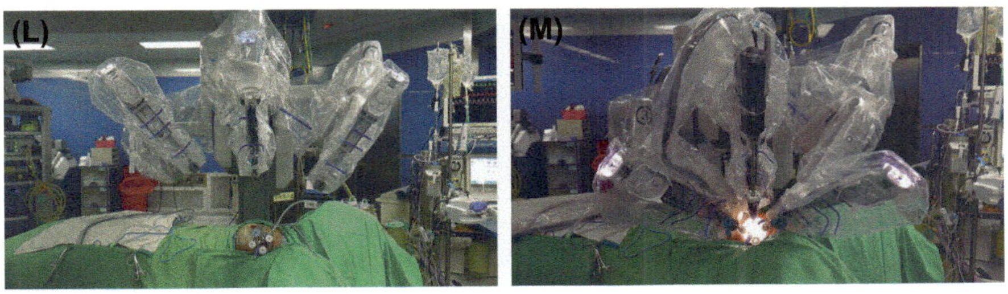

10.22L, M

Operating theater view showing the intra-operative setting, which was performed with a da Vinci Si (Intuitive Surgical, Sunnyvale, CA) robotic platform with the operating surgeon controlling at the surgeon's console.

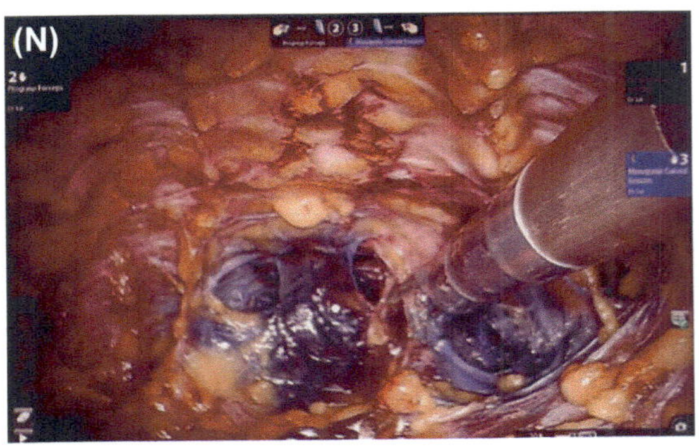

10.22N

Dissection of skin flap with monopolar scissors.

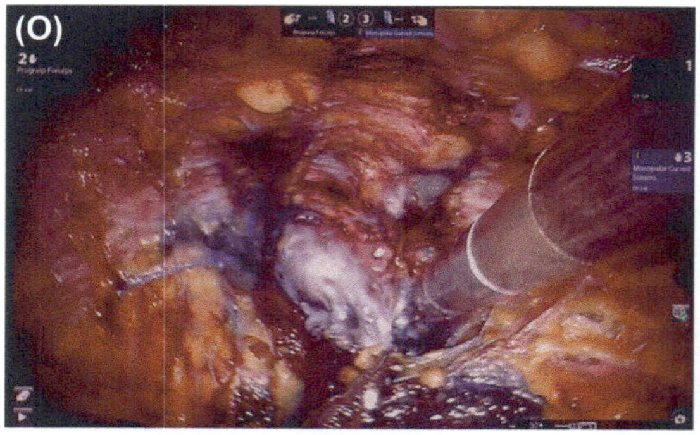

10.22O

Intra-operative sub-nipple biopsies performed for the frozen section analysis.

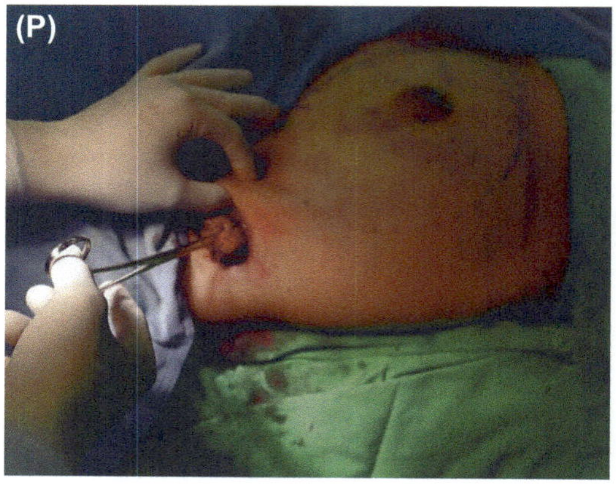

10.22P

Specimen removed via axillary incision.

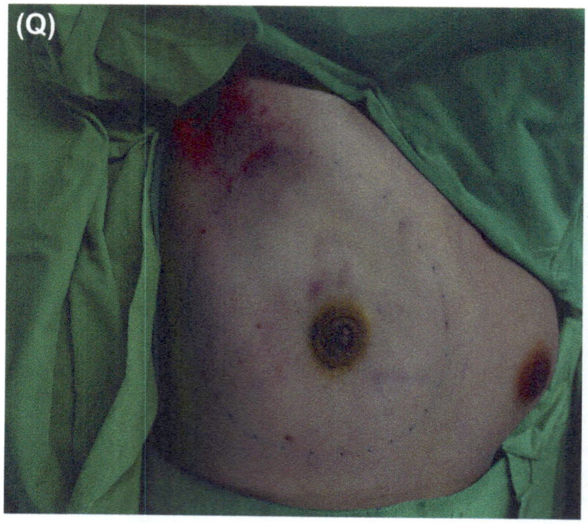

10.22Q

Immediate on table view after mastectomy and removal of single port.

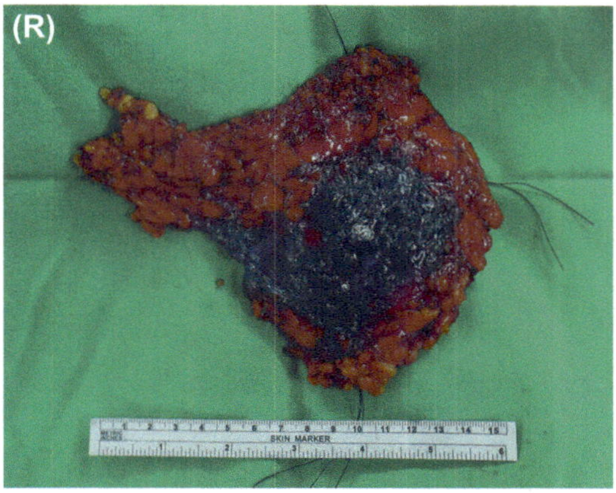

10.22R

Mastectomy specimen removed intact and oriented.

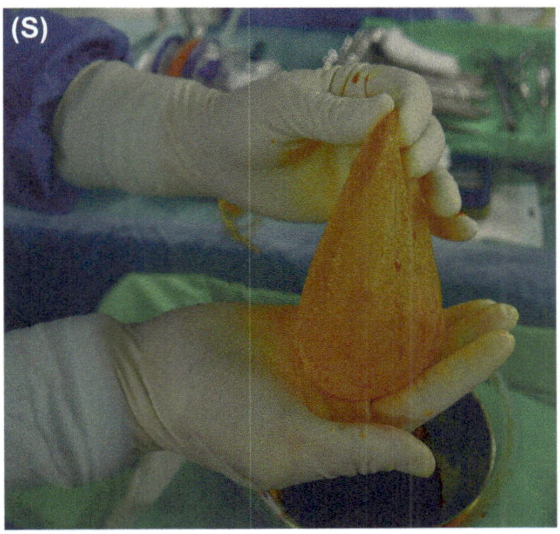

10.22S

Gel implant.

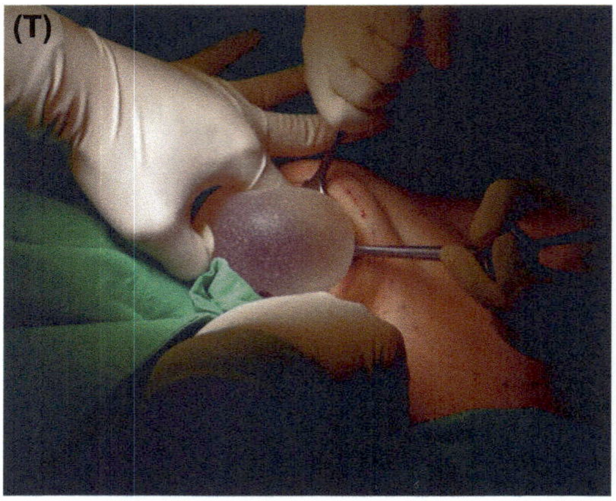

10.22T

Gel implant was inserted from the axillary incision and placed in the submuscular pocket.

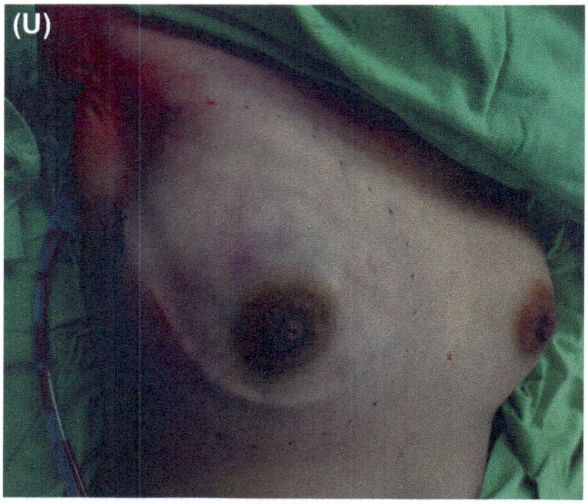

10.22U

Immediate on-table view after wound closure.

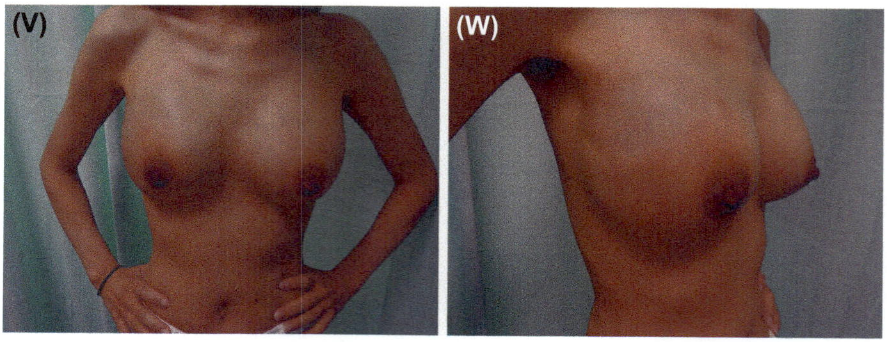

10.22V, W

6 months post-operative views showing excellent cosmesis and symmetry.

Case 23: Bilateral robotic nipple-sparing mastectomy with immediate implant reconstruction – single incision

Patient/Demographics

The case described a 37-year-old lady who initially presented after an abnormal screening mammogram in her right breast and a stereotactic-guided vacuum-assisted biopsy revealed ductal carcinoma in situ. A genetic counseling and testing were performed which did not reveal any mutation or carrier status to suggest hereditary breast cancer.

She was keen for risk-reducing mastectomy for the contralateral side and decided for robotic nipple-sparing mastectomy with immediate implant reconstruction.

Surgery and pathology report

Patient underwent bilateral robotic nipple-sparing mastectomy with right sentinel lymph node biopsy and immediate implant reconstruction. Intra-operative frozen section for right sentinel lymph node and bilateral sub-nipple biopsies was negative.

Her final histology reported TisN0M0 (Stage 0) disease, and she did not receive any adjuvant therapy thereafter.

Post-operative outcomes

Patient was discharged 5 days after her operation with an uneventful post-operative recovery thereafter. Patient was reviewed at regular intervals after operation and graded her post-operative cosmesis as excellent.

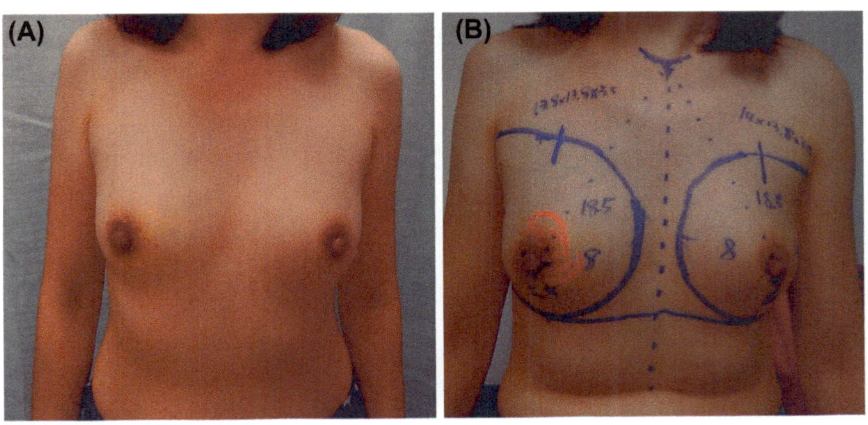

10.23A, 10.23B

Pre-operative front views with markings showing tumor location.

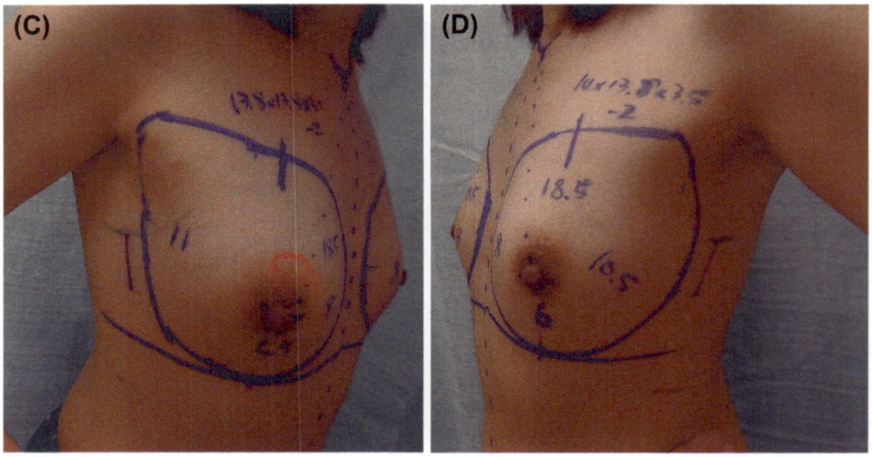

10.23C, 10.23D

Pre-op views showing planned incision along anterior axillary line.

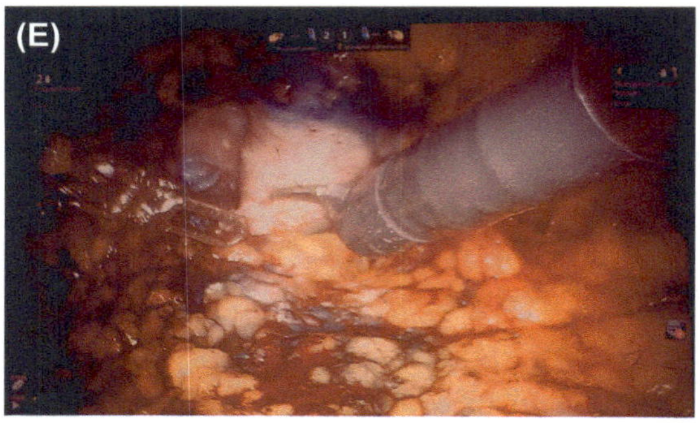

10.23E

Intra-operative sub-nipple biopsies performed for frozen section analysis.

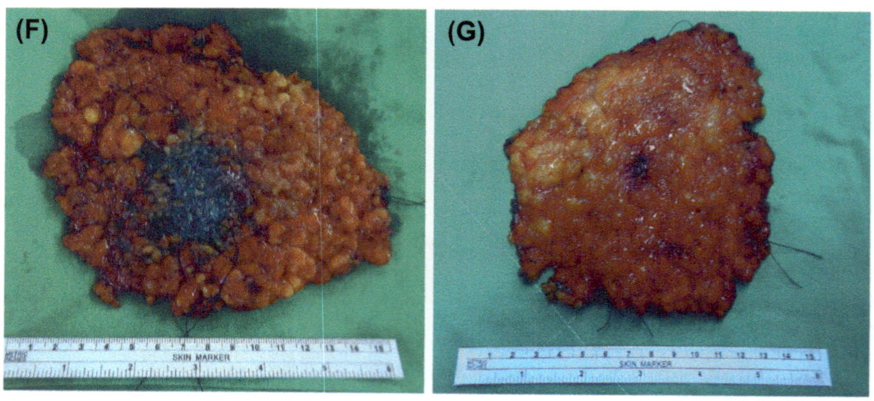

10.23F, 10.23G

Bilateral mastectomy specimens removed intact and oriented.

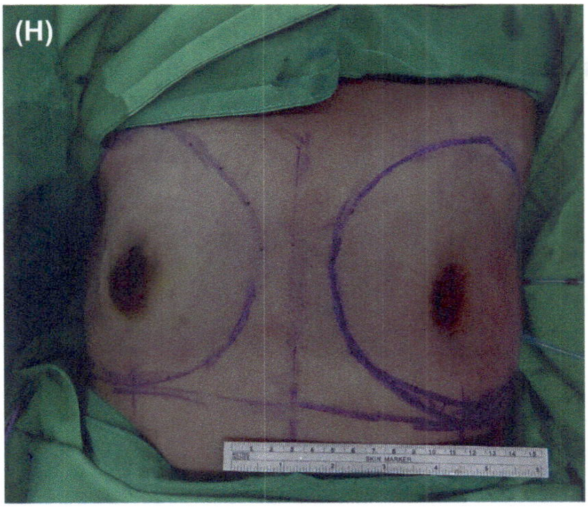

10.23H

Immediate on-table view after mastectomy and removal of single port.

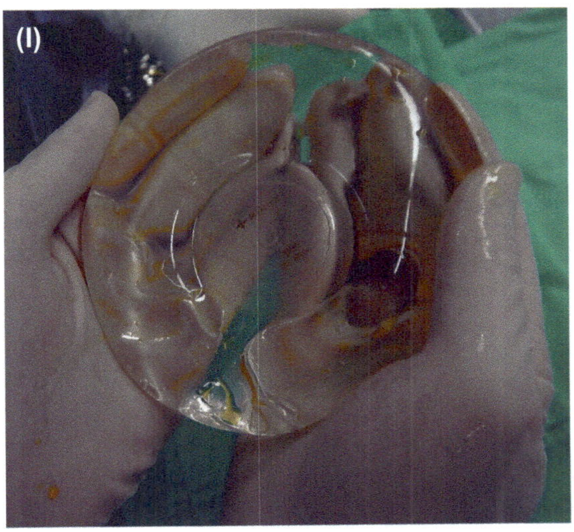

10.23I

Gel implant of appropriate volume and size were selected and placed in the submuscular pocket from the axillary incision.

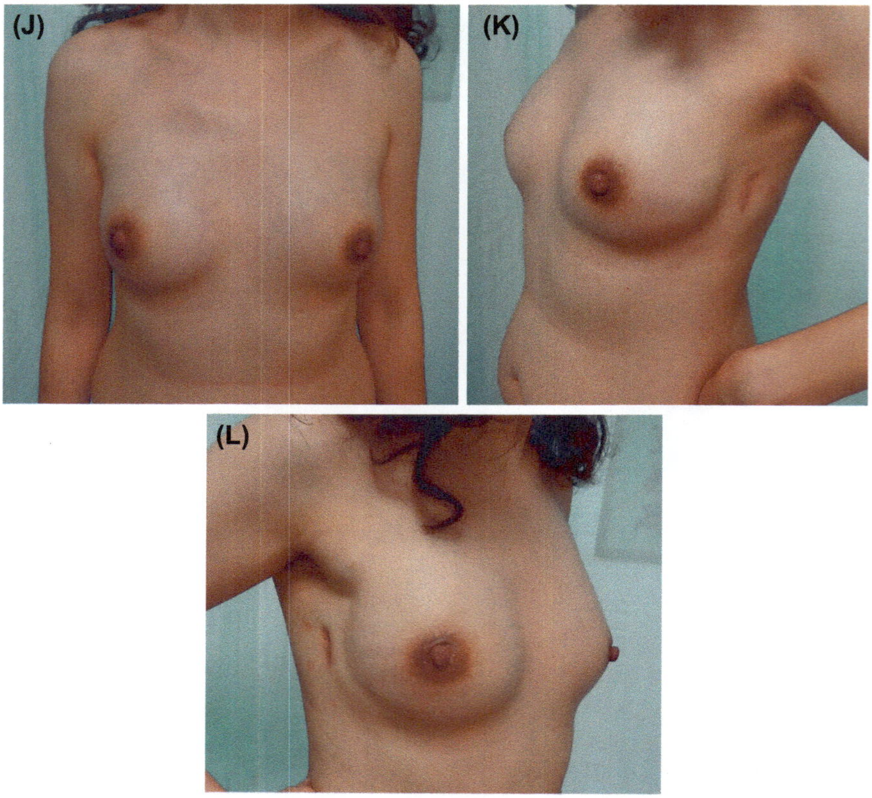

10.23J, 10.23K, 10.23L

3 months post-operative views showing excellent cosmesis and symmetry.

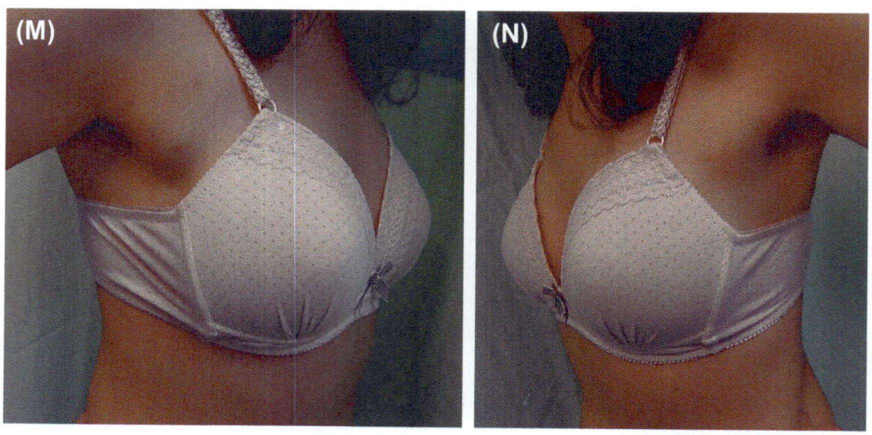

10.23M, 10.23N

3 months post-operative views showing hidden incisions along bra line.

Case 24: Robotic nipple-sparing mastectomy with immediate implant reconstruction – single axillary incision, da Vinci Xi system

Patient/Demographics

The case described a 55-year-old lady diagnosed with a clinical Stage I left breast cancer with a pre-operative core biopsy report of an invasive ductal carcinoma with ductal carcinoma in situ, ER/PR +, and CerbB2+. Her metastatic workup did not reveal any distant metastases.

After extensive counseling, patient decided for a robotic nipple-sparing mastectomy with immediate implant reconstruction.

Surgery and pathology report

Patient underwent a left robotic nipple-sparing mastectomy with sentinel lymph node biopsy and immediate implant reconstruction. Intra-operative frozen section for sentinel lymph node and sub-nipple biopsies was negative.

Her final histology reported a T1aN0M0 (Stage IA) disease, and she was counseled for 5 years of adjuvant endocrine therapy thereafter.

Post-operative outcomes

She was discharged 4 days after her initial operation with an uneventful post-operative recovery thereafter. Patient was reviewed at regular intervals after operation, and her post-operative cosmesis was graded as excellent.

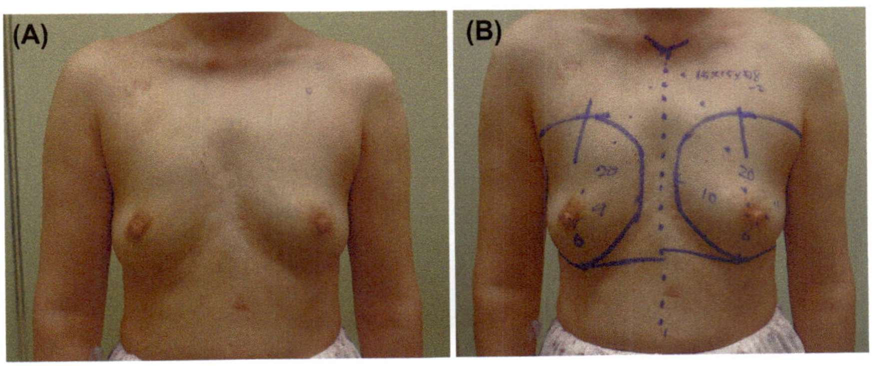

10.24A, 10.24B

Pre-operative front views with pre-operative markings as shown.

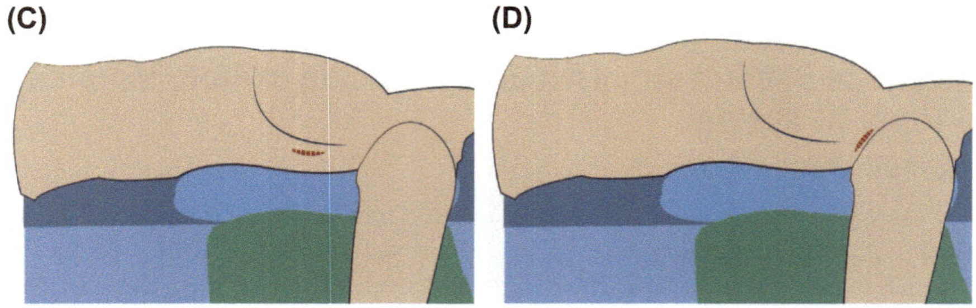

10.24C, 10.24D

Graphic illustrations depicting common incisions used for robotic nipple sparing mastectomy, along anterior axillary line (Figure 10.24c) and axillary incision (Figure 10.24d).

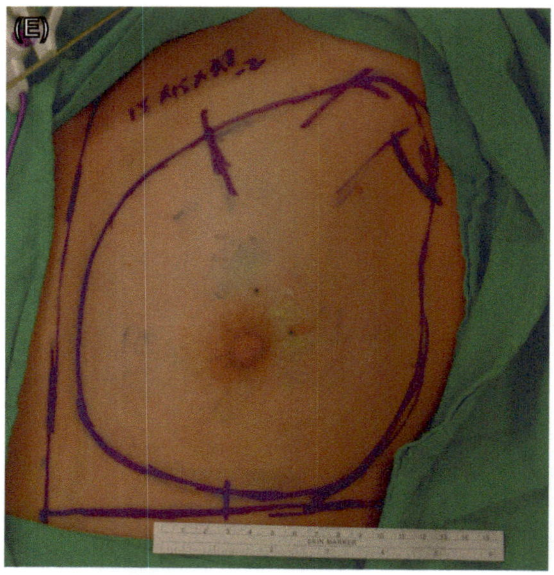

10.24E

On-table view showing marking of resection boundaries as well as planned axillary incision.

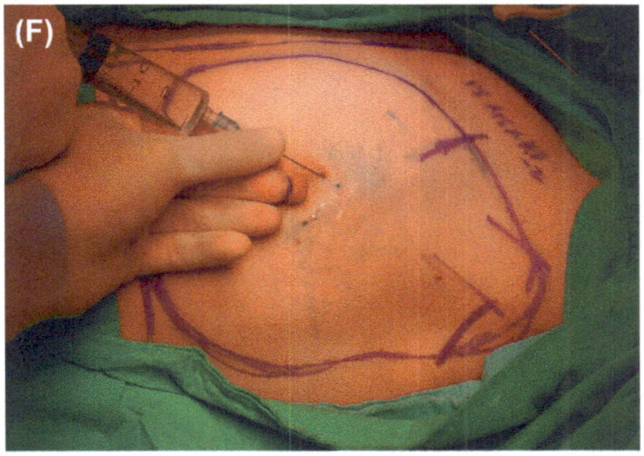

10.24F

A physiological saline solution containing lidocaine 0.05% and epinephrine 1:1,000,000 was injected subcutaneously into the whole breast to minimize bleeding.

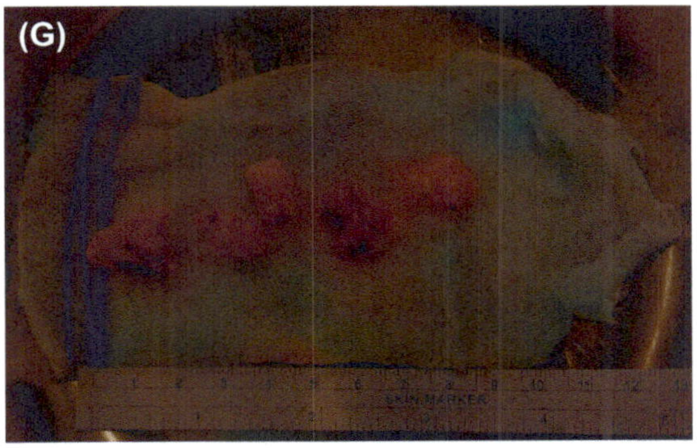

10.24G

Sentinel lymph nodes retrieved and sent for intra-operative frozen section analysis.

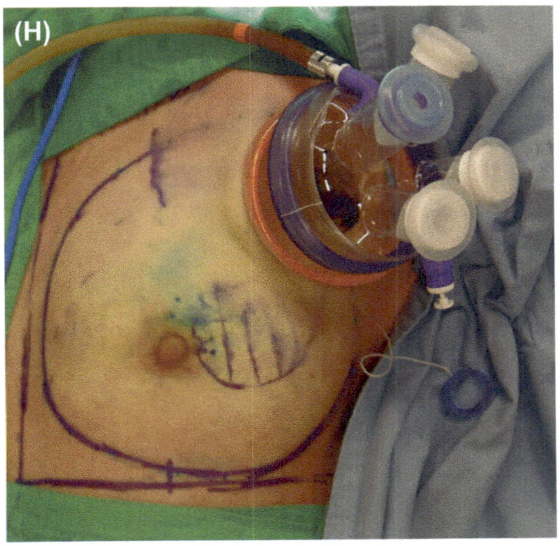

10.24H

After creation of the working space, a single port (Glove Port, Nelis, Gyeonggi-do, Korea) was placed with CO_2 insufflation to 8mmHg.

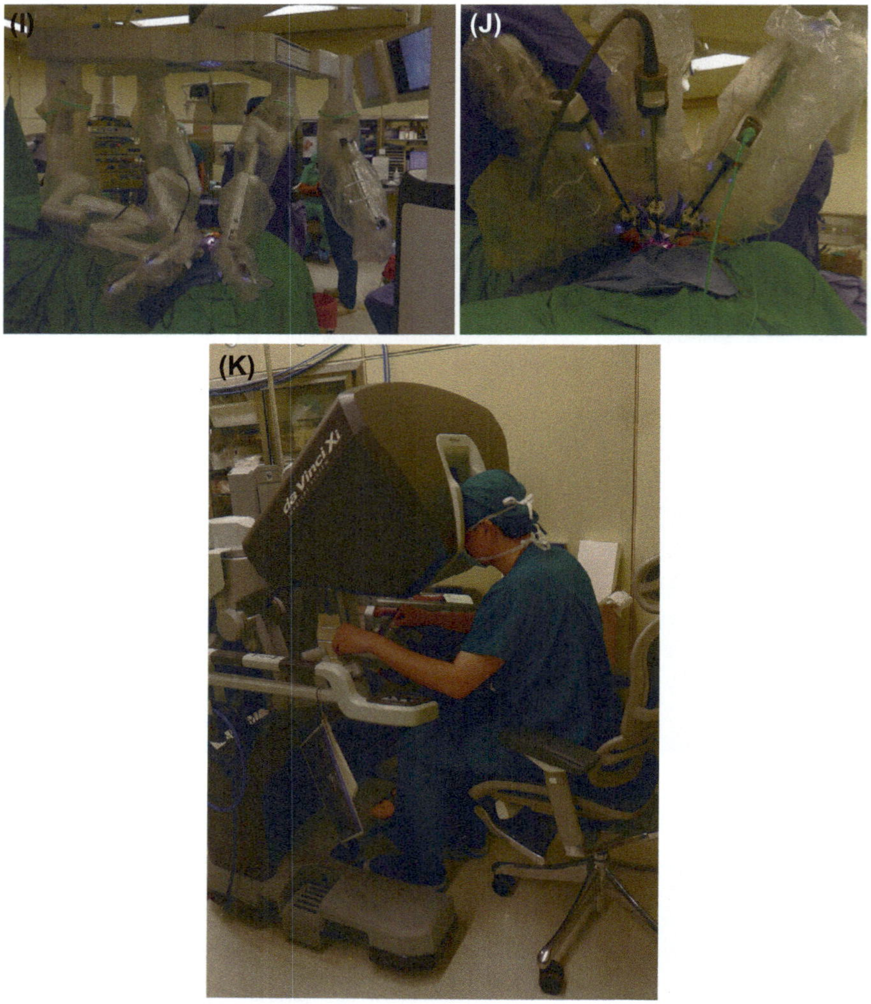

10.24I, 10.24J, 10.24K

Operating-theater view showing the intra-operative setting, which was performed with a da Vinci Xi (Intuitive Surgical, Sunnyvale, CA) robotic platform with the operating surgeon controlling at the surgeon's console.

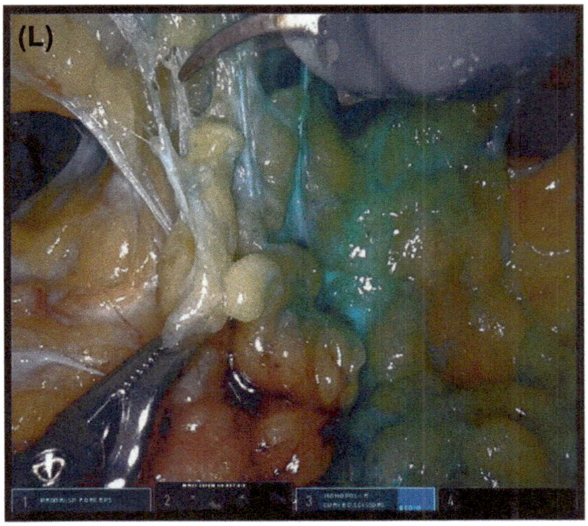

10.24L

Dissection of skin flap with monopolar scissors.

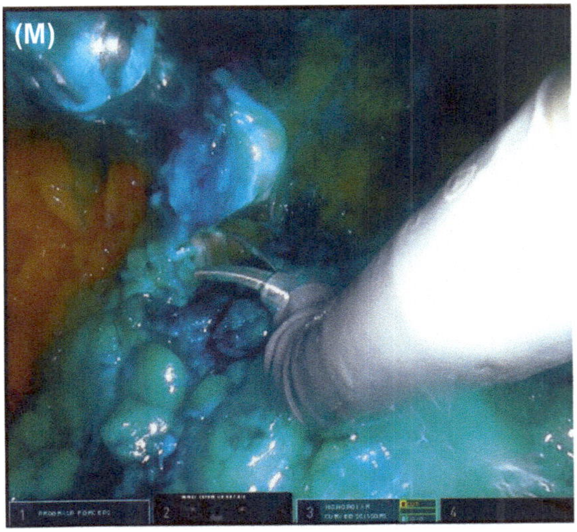

10.24M

Intra-operative sub-nipple biopsies performed for frozen section analysis.

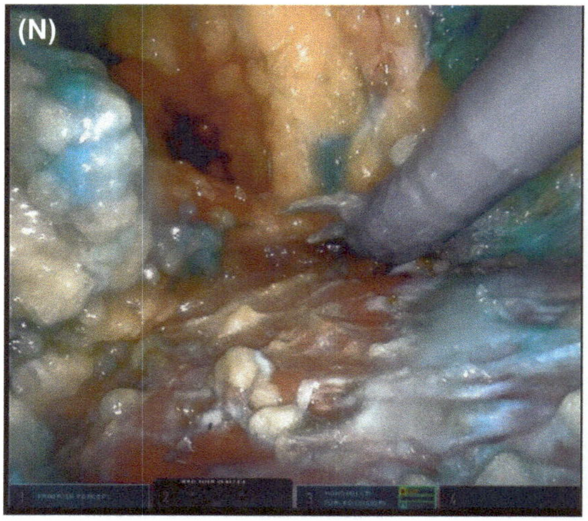

10.24N

Peripheral and posterior dissection of breast parenchyma off pectoralis major fascia.

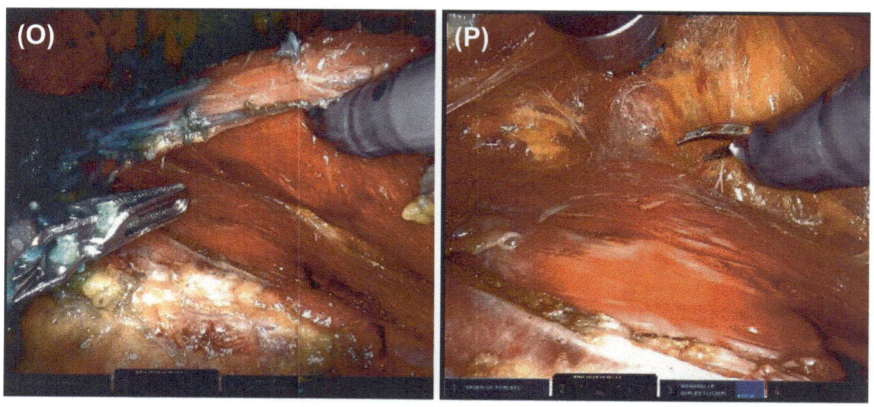

10.24O, 10.24P

Dissection and development of submuscular pocket for subsequent implant placement.

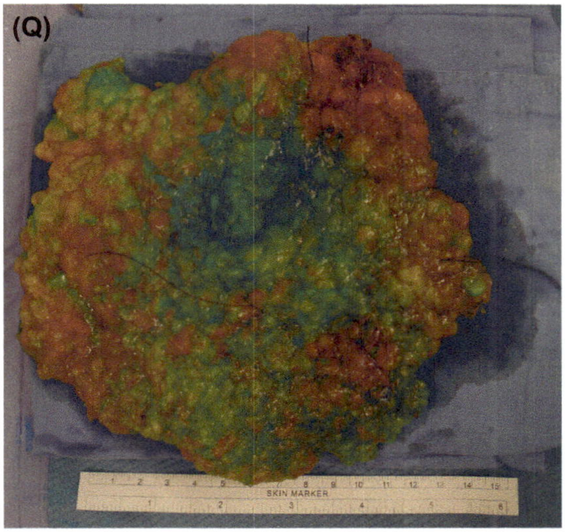

10.24Q

Mastectomy specimen removed in entirety via axillary incision and oriented.

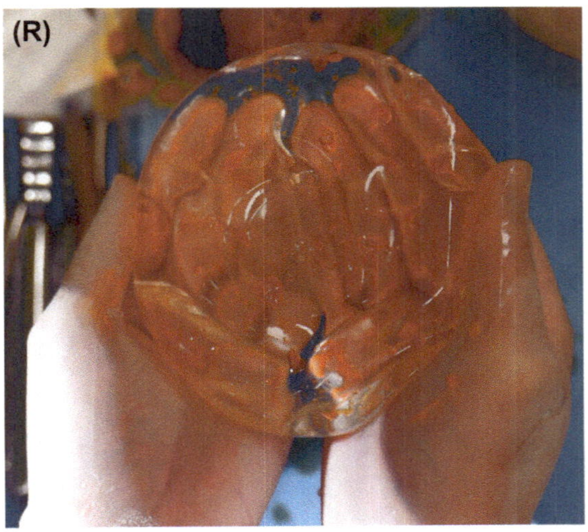

10.24R

Gel implant of appropriate volume and size chosen and placed in the subpectoral plane via the axillary incision.

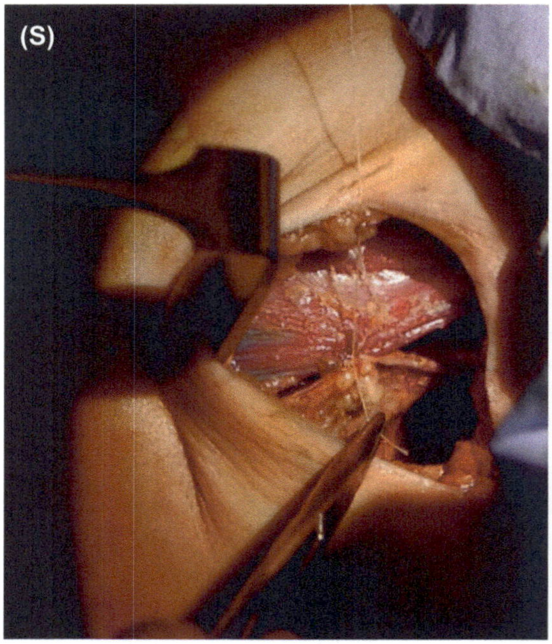

10.24S

Lateral border of pectoralis major tagged to serratus anterior to hold implant and avoid lateral migration of implant.

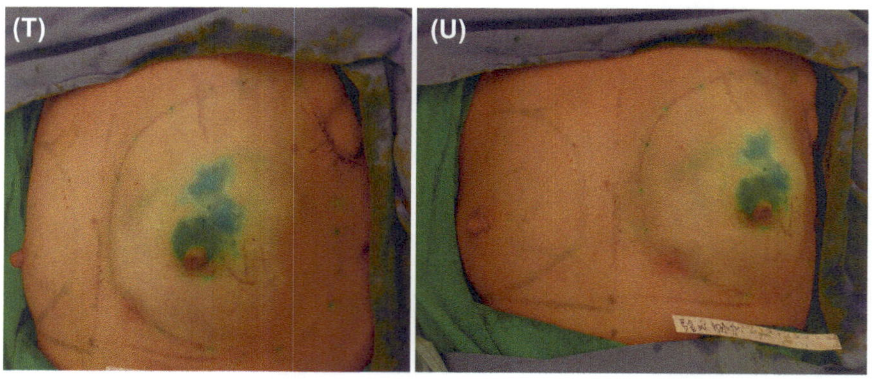

10.24T, 10.24U

Immediate on-table views after wound closure.

Case 25: Robotic nipple-sparing mastectomy with immediate implant reconstruction – single incision, da Vinci Si system

Patient/Demographics

The case described a 51-year-old lady diagnosed with left breast malignancy with a pre-operative core biopsy report of an invasive ductal carcinoma, ER/PR +, and CerbB2 negative.

Her metastatic workup did not reveal any distant metastases.

Patient decided for a left robotic nipple-sparing mastectomy and sentinel lymph node biopsy with immediate implant reconstruction.

Surgery and pathology report

Patient underwent a left robotic nipple-sparing mastectomy with sentinel lymph node biopsy and immediate implant reconstruction. Intra-operative frozen section for sentinel lymph node and sub-nipple biopsies was negative.

Her final histology reported T1cN1micM0 (Stage IB) disease, and she was counseled for adjuvant chemotherapy followed by 5 years of endocrine therapy.

Post-operative outcomes

She was discharged 4 days after her operation with an uneventful post-operative recovery thereafter. Patient was reviewed at regular intervals after operation, and her post-operative cosmesis was graded as excellent.

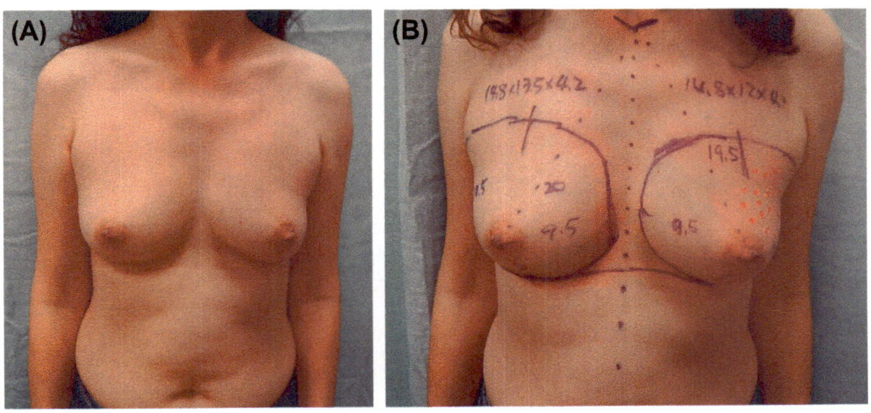

10.25A, 10.25B

Pre-operative front views with markings showing tumor location.

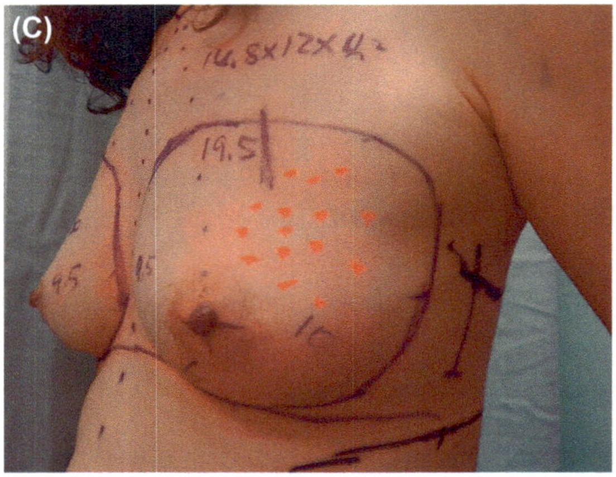

10.25C

Pre-operative lateral view showing planned incision along anterior axillary line.

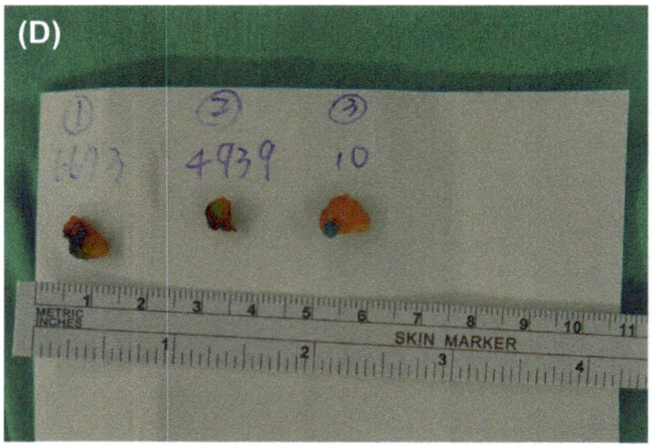

10.25D

Sentinel lymph nodes identified using dual modality were retrieved and sent for intra-operative frozen section analysis.

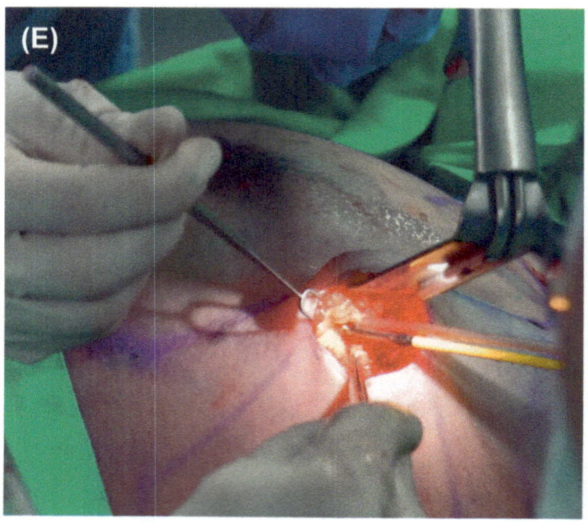

10.25E

Dissection and creation of working space before placement of single port.

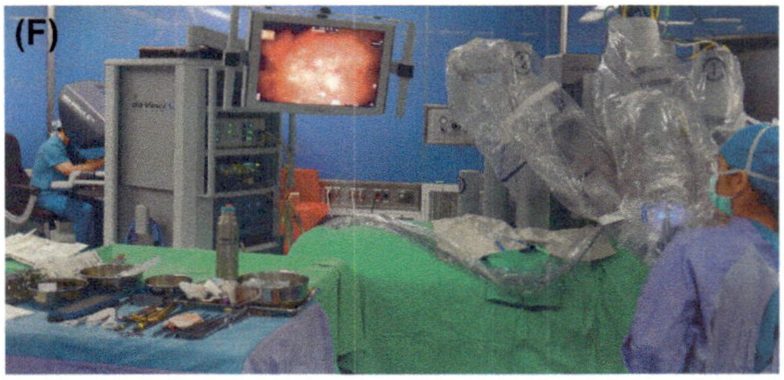

10.25F

Operating theater view showing the intra-operative setting, which was performed with a da Vinci Si (Intuitive Surgical, Sunnyvale, CA) robotic platform with the operating surgeon controlling at the surgeon's console.

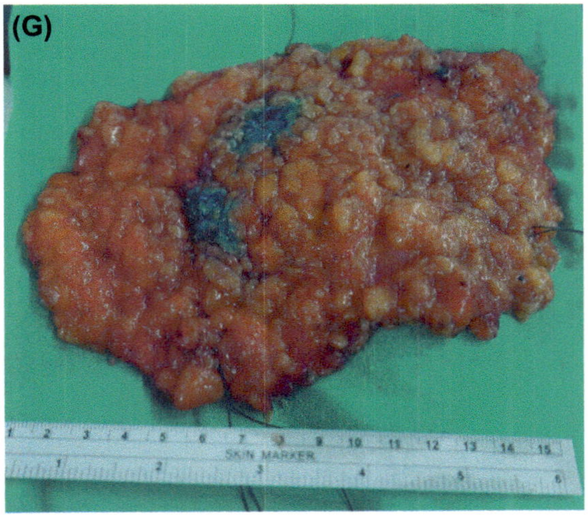

10.25G

Mastectomy specimen removed intact and oriented.

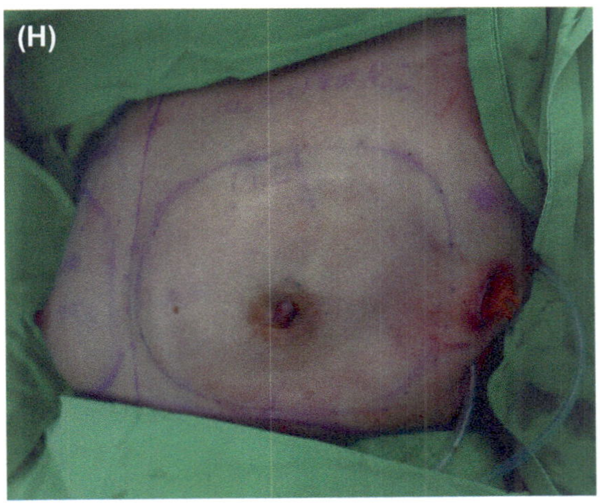

10.25H

Immediate on-table view after mastectomy and removal of robotic arms.

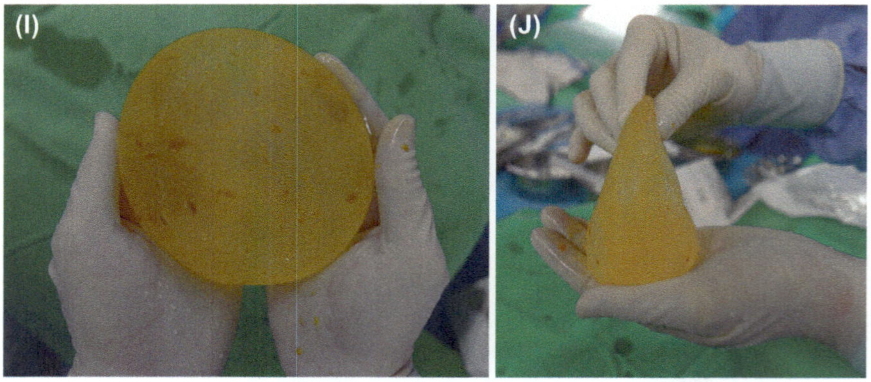

10.25I, 10.25J

Gel implant of appropriate size and volume was chosen and placed in the submuscular pocket through the axillary incision.

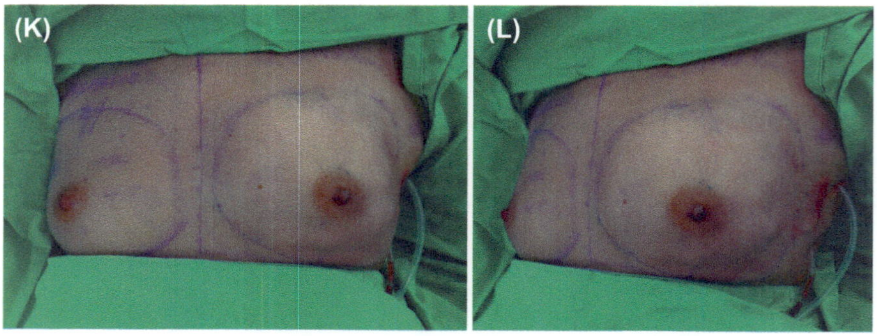

10.25K, 10.25L

Immediate on-table views after wound closure.

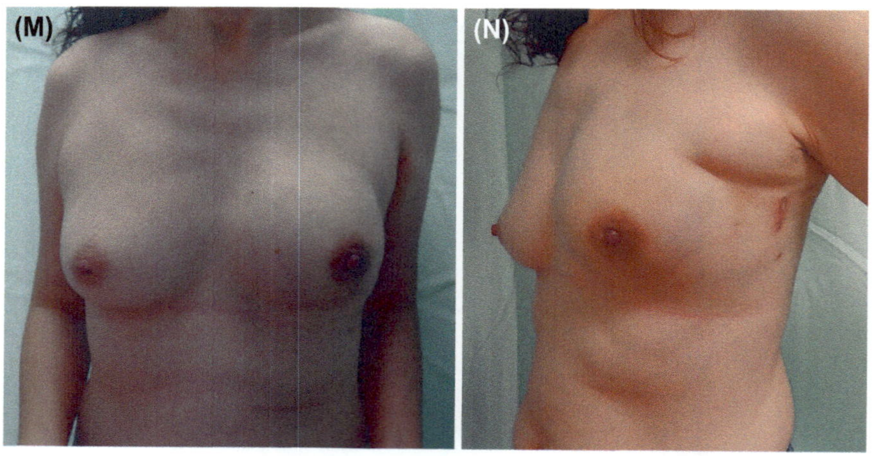

10.25M, 10.25N

1 month post-operative views showing excellent cosmesis.

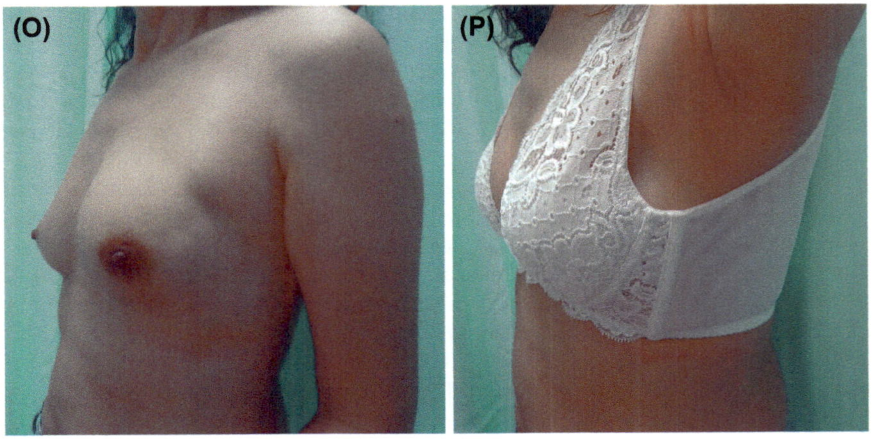

10.25O, 10.25P

Lateral views showing incision well hidden along anterior axillary and bra line.

Discussion

Due to high patient satisfaction rates and acceptable oncologic safety, NSM was increasingly performed in patients with breast cancer without apparent NAC invasion (Mallon et al., 2013). R-NSM via da Vinci surgical platform enables the operation to be performed through small and inconspicuous extra-mammary axillary wound. The cosmetic outcome in preliminary studies (Sarfati et al., 2018; Toesca et al., 2017; Lai et al., 2018; Lai et al., 2019) were good and could therefore be a promising new technique for patients indicated for nipple-sparing mastectomy who desire a small and inconspicuous scar. From technical feasibility point of view, the strength of this innovative surgical technique lies in the fact that it addresses the technical difficulty in endoscopic nipple-sparing mastectomy (E-NSM) as the conventional rigid endoscopic instruments were inferior to the more flexible instruments in R-NSM. Second, endoscopic approach requires an assistant to hold and control the camera compared to R-NSM whereby the need for assistance is obviated, hence potentially enabling an easier and more ergonomic surgical solution (Lai et al., 2019). The drawback with the application of R-NSM as it is with other procedures utilizing da Vinci surgical platform, will be the cost involved.

References

Lai, H. W., Lin, S. L., Chen, S. T., Chen, S. L., Lin, Y. L., Chen, D. R., & Kuo, S. J. (2018). Robotic Nipple-sparing Mastectomy and Immediate Breast Reconstruction with Gel Implant. *Plast Reconstr Surg Glob Open*, *6*(6), e1828. https://doi.org/10.1097/GOX.0000000000001828. eCollection 2018 Jun. PMID:30276055. https://www.ncbi.nlm.nih.gov/pubmed/30276055

Lai, H. W., Wang, C. C., Lai, Y. C., Chen, C. J., Lin, S. L., Chen, S. T., Lin, Y. J., Chen, D. R., & Kuo, S. J. (2019). The learning curve of robotic nipple sparing mastectomy for breast cancer: An analysis of consecutive 39 procedures with cumulative sum plot. *European Journal of Surgical Oncology, 45*(2), 125–133. https://doi.org/10.1016/j.ejso.2018.09.021. Epub 2018 Oct 17. PMID:30360987. https://www.ncbi.nlm.nih.gov/pubmed/30360987

Lai, H. W., et al. (2019). Robotic Nipple-Sparing mastectomy and immediate breast reconstruction with Gel implant: technique, preliminary results and patient-reported cosmetic outcome. *Annals of Surgical Oncology, 26*(1), 42–52.

Mallon, P., Feron, J. G., Couturaud, B., Fitoussi, A., Lemasurier, P., Guihard, T., et al. (2013). The role of nipple-sparing mastectomy in breast cancer: A comprehensive review of the literature. *Plastic and Reconstructive Surgery.* https://doi.org/10.1097/PRS.0b013e3182865a3c.

Sarfati, B., Struk, S., Leymarie, N., Honart, J. F., Alkhashnam, H., Tran de Fremicourt, K., et al. (2018). Robotic prophylactic nipple-sparing mastectomy with immediate prosthetic breast reconstruction: A prospective study. *Annals of Surgical Oncology.* https://doi.org/10.1245/s10434-018-6555-x.

Toesca, A., Peradze, N., Manconi, A., Galimberti, V., Intra, M., Colleoni, M., et al. (2017). Robotic nipple-sparing mastectomy for the treatment of breast cancer: Feasibility and safety study. *Breast.* https://doi.org/10.1016/j.breast.2016.10.009.

CHAPTER

Robotic mastectomy with immediate latissimus dorsi flap reconstruction

11

Description of technique

Pre-operative marking and positioning

Pre-operative marking was done with the patient in standing and supine position. After induction of general anaesthesia, the patient was then placed in the supine position and ipsilateral arm abducted to 90 degrees to avoid affecting the operative procedure.

Axillary staging procedure

In patients for whom sentinel lymph node biopsy (SLNB) is indicated, a small amount (2–3 mCi) of radioisotope Tc99m was injected intradermally at the site of the tumour before operation (either on the day or 1 day prior).

After induction of general anaesthesia, 3 mL of 1% methylene blue (Merck, Darmstadt, Germany) was injected into the breast parenchyma in equally divided aliquots at five positions surrounding the hemisphere of the tumour facing the ipsilateral axilla. The breast tissue from the tumour to the axilla was then gently massaged for 5–10 minutes. Within 20–30 minutes after injection of the blue dye, a handheld gamma probe (Navigator; USSC, Norwalk, CT) was used to identify the hot spots and the location of the hottest nodes was then marked. An approximately 3–5 cm oblique axillary incision was then made close to the hottest nodes and SLNB was then performed. Fresh frozen section was performed as indicated. If SLN was positive for metastases, a complete axillary lymph node dissection up to level II was performed.

Robotic docking and dissection

To create working space for placement of the single port (Glove Port; Nelis Corporation, Gyeonggi-do, Korea), a 3–4 cm subcutaneous flap was dissected with electrocautery under direct vision. The tunnelling technique as described in

Minimally Invasive (Endoscopic & Robotic) Breast Surgery. https://doi.org/10.1016/B978-0-323-73405-9.00011-X

endoscopic mastectomy was then used to facilitate skin flap dissection and create space between the skin flap and the breast parenchyma. Once adequate dissection was achieved, the single port was then inserted through the axilla incision, and carbon dioxide (CO_2) insufflation with air pressure kept at 8 mmHg was used to create space for mastectomy. The ipsilateral shoulder was elevated to 30 degrees to prevent conflict between the operating table and docking of the robotic surgery system. The robotic side cart (da Vinci; Intuitive Surgical, Sunnyvale, CA, USA) was then positioned from the contralateral side, with the two robotic arms endoscope extending over the patient near the ports before the ports were docked to the robotic arms. Subsequently, the operation was then shifted to the da Vinci Si or Xi (Intuitive Surgical, Sunnyvale, CA, USA) robotic platform controlled by the operating surgeon at the console. The authors used a 30-degree 12-mm diameter camera (Intuitive Surgical, Denzlingen, Germany) in the upper port to prevent collisions with other instruments. Dissection was carried out using an 8-mm monopolar scissors (Intuitive Surgical, Sunnyvale, CA, USA). Traction and counter-traction, along with maintaining exposure, was carried out using an 8 mm ProGrasp forceps (Intuitive Surgical, Sunnyvale, CA, USA). The location of the scissors and the ProGrasp forceps could be changed inter-variably during the operation. Dissection was initiated from the superficial skin flaps by dissecting the septa between the skin flap and parenchyma created by the tunnelling technique with monopolar scissors. A sub-nipple biopsy and fresh frozen section analysis can be performed in a nipple-sparing mastectomy. If cancer cell invasion was found in the sub-areolar area, the entire nipple-areola complex was removed and conversion to a skin-sparing mastectomy was then performed. After completion of the superficial skin flap dissection, dissection of the peripheral portion of the breast parenchyma was carried out subsequently. Posterior dissection was then performed by detaching the breast tissue from the pectoralis major muscle fascia with the perforator vessels clearly identified and secured. After completion of dissection, the entire breast specimen was removed through the axillary wound.

Immediate pedicled latissimus dorsi flap reconstruction

Following removal of the specimen and adequate haemostasis, copious irrigation of the mastectomy pocket was performed. Subsequently, the thoracodorsal pedicle was identified and marked with a vessel loop to prevent injury during the flap harvest. Patient was then shifted to the lateral decubitus position. Two 12 mm balloon trocars (Kii Balloon blunt tip system, Applied Medical, Rancho Santa Margarita, CA, USA) were used as working ports. The ports were then docked to the robotic arms, and CO_2 insufflation was applied at

10–12 mmHg. Dissection was started along the under surface of the latissimus dorsi (LD) muscle. Blood vessels encountered were carefully dissected, coagulated and cut with monopolar scissors. As the dissection through the under surface of the muscle to the borders was completed, further dissection over the superficial surface of the muscle ensued. The muscle was disconnected from the infero-posterior and scapular border. Afterwards, the pedicled LD flap was exteriorized from the axilla wound and the robotic arms were then undocked. Reconstruction of the mastectomy defect was performed with the patient turned back to a supine position. Fixation of the flap to all quadrants was performed with assistance from a handle light retractor to ensure full coverage of the defect. Care must be taken to ensure the correct axis of the vascular pedicle to prevent torsion of the blood supply. Drains were then placed both in the donor site and in the mastectomy cavity.

Case 26: robotic nipple-sparing mastectomy with immediate pedicled latissimus dorsi flap reconstruction

Patient/demographics

The patient is a 49-year-old lady who presented with an excision biopsy of a left breast lump in another institution which was reported as lobular carcinoma in situ with involved margins. She did not have any palpable lumps in both breasts except for a periareolar scar in her left breast.

Her metastatic workup was not performed in view of excision biopsy histology.

She was keen for mastectomy with reconstruction and was therefore offered robotic nipple-sparing mastectomy, sentinel lymph node biopsy with immediate pedicled latissimus dorsi (LD) reconstruction.

Surgery and pathology report

This lady underwent a left robotic nipple sparing mastectomy with immediate pedicled LD reconstruction. Sentinel lymph node and sub-nipple biopsies for the frozen section analysis were negative. Her final histology reported residual LCIS, TisN0M0, stage 0 disease and therefore did not receive any adjuvant therapy.

Post-operative outcomes

No immediate post-operative complications were encountered. The patient was reviewed at regular intervals in outpatient clinic and reported high satisfaction over her post-op cosmesis.

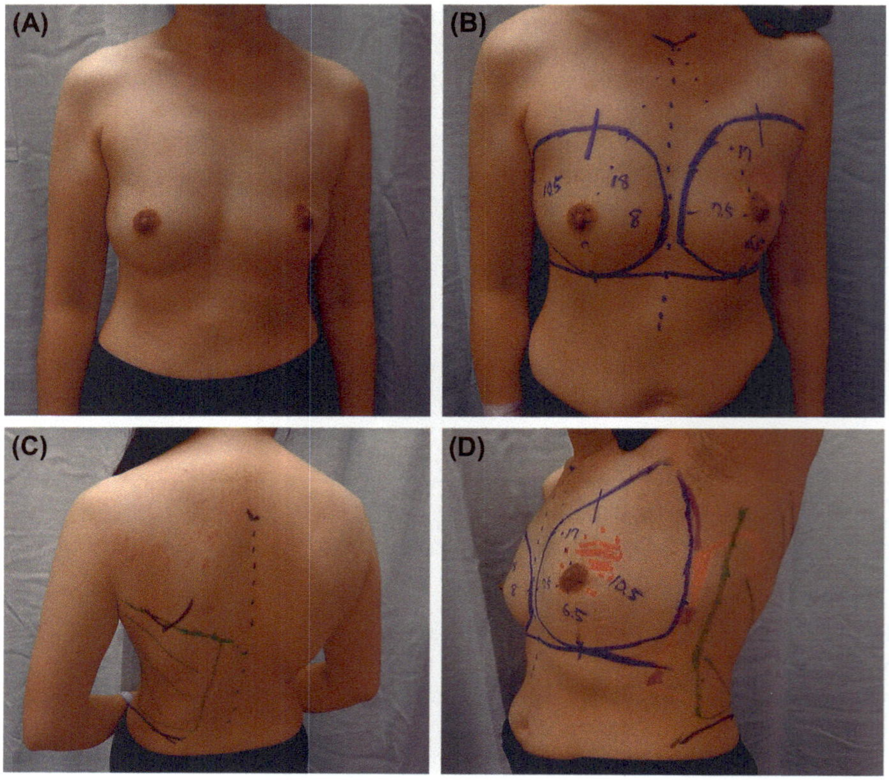

11.26A–D

Pre-operative views with markings showing tumor location, planned incisions, as well as markings for latissimus dorsi (LD) flap.

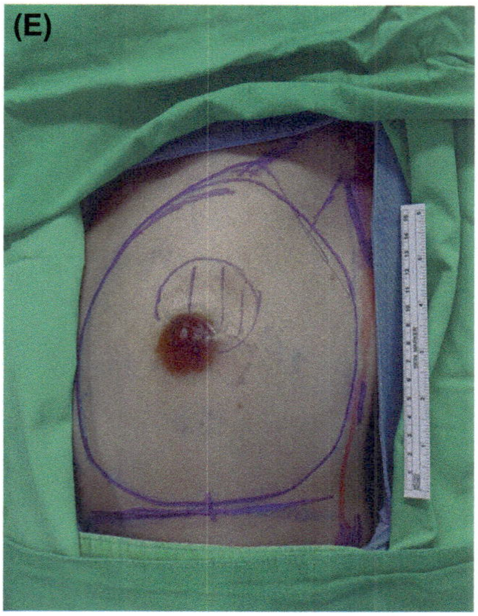

11.26E

On-table view showing planned incisions.

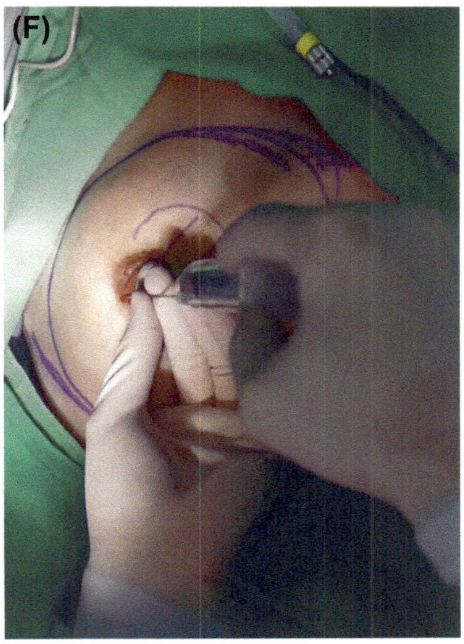

11.26F

A physiological saline solution containing lidocaine 0.05% and epinephrine 1:1,000,000 was injected subcutaneously into the whole breast to minimize bleeding.

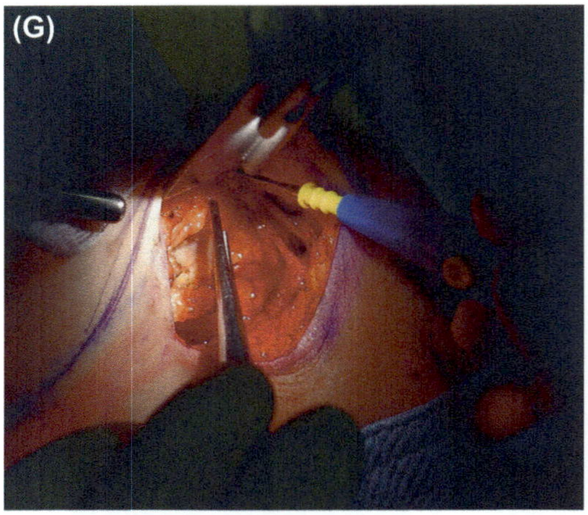

11.26G

Sentinel lymph node biopsy performed via axillary incision.

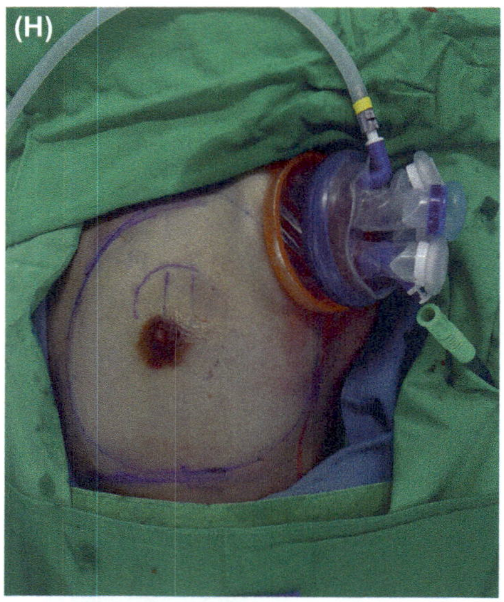

11.26H

After sentinel lymph node biopsy and creation of adequate working space, a single port (Glove Port, Nelis, Gyeonggi-do, Korea) was placed with CO_2 insufflation to 8 mmHg.

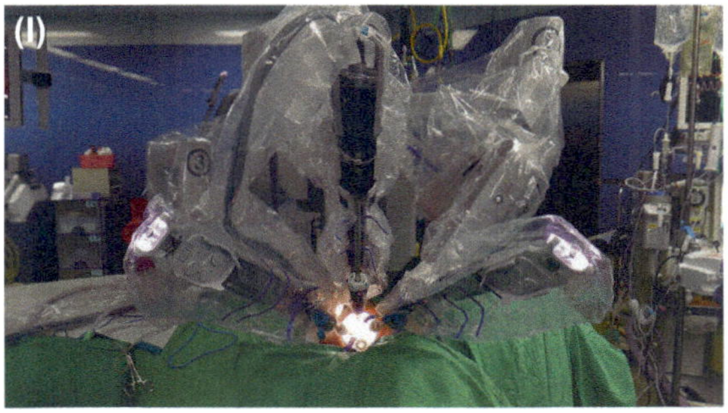

11.26I

Operating theater view showing the intra-operative setting, which was performed with a da Vinci Si (Intuitive Surgical, Sunnyvale, CA) robotic platform with the operating surgeon controlling at the surgeon's console.

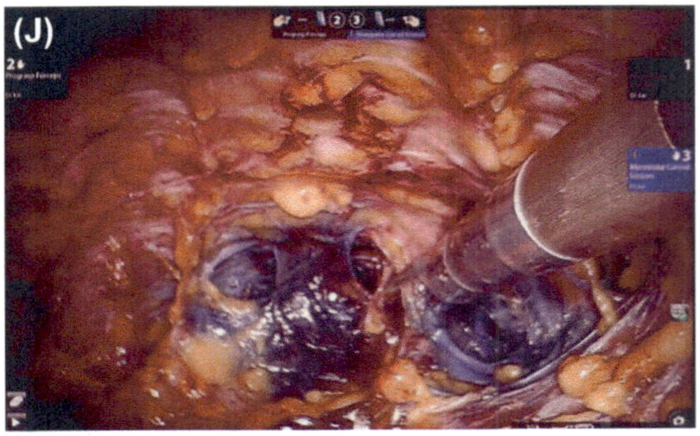

11.26J

Dissection of skin flap with monopolar scissors.

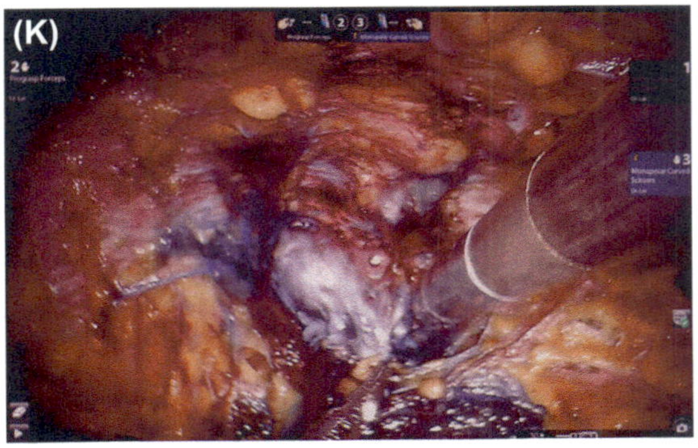

11.26K

Intra-operative sub-nipple biopsies performed for the frozen section analysis.

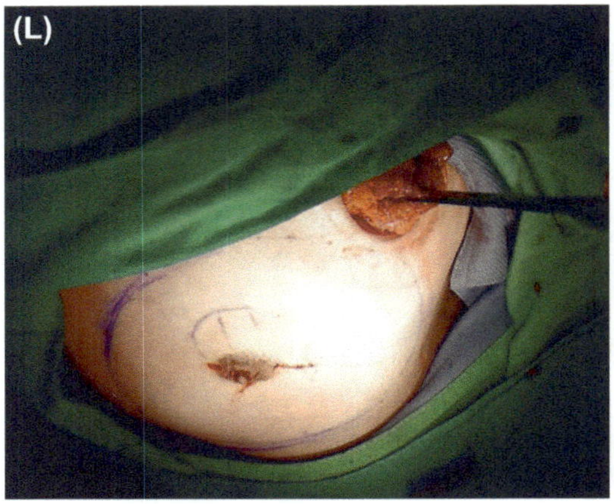

11.26L

Specimen removed via axillary incision.

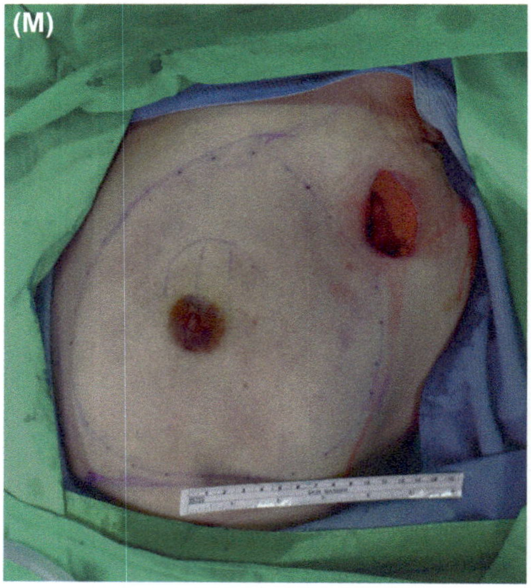

11.26M

Immediate on-table view after mastectomy and removal of single port.

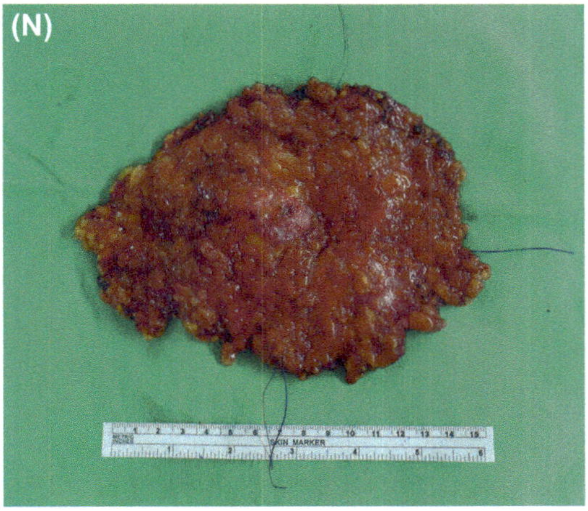

11.26N

Mastectomy specimen removed intact and oriented.

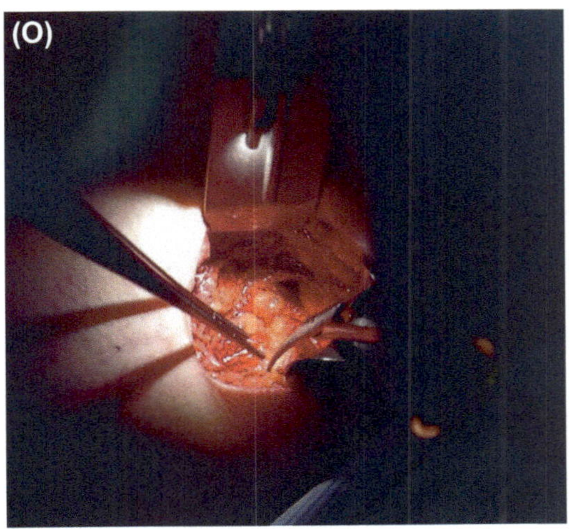

11.26O

Dissection of axilla and isolation of thoracodorsal bundle before LD flap harvest.

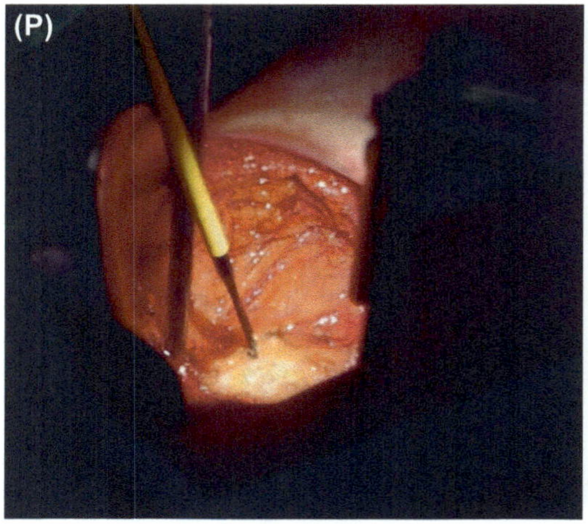

11.26P

Creation of adequate working space before re-positioning and harvest of flap.

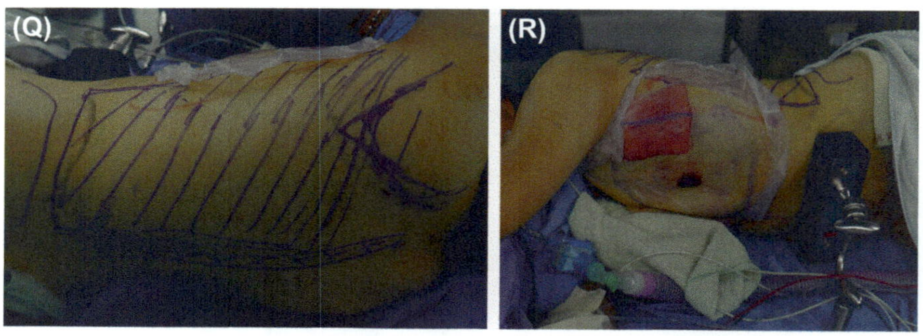

11.26Q, R

Patient positioned to lateral decubitus position in preparation for robotic-assisted LD flap harvest.

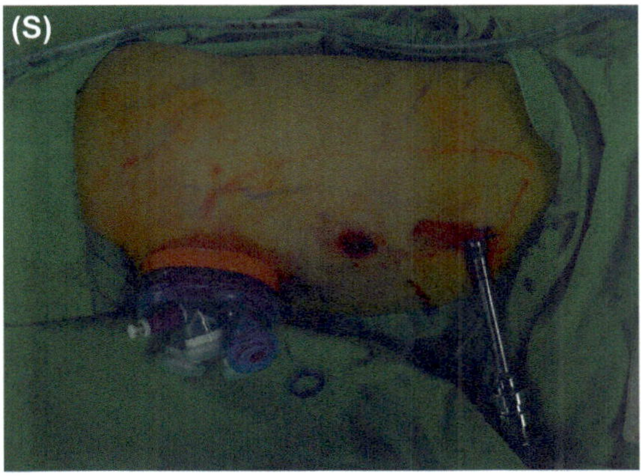

11.26S

Single port and two additional 12 mm working ports were placed before docking of robotic arms.

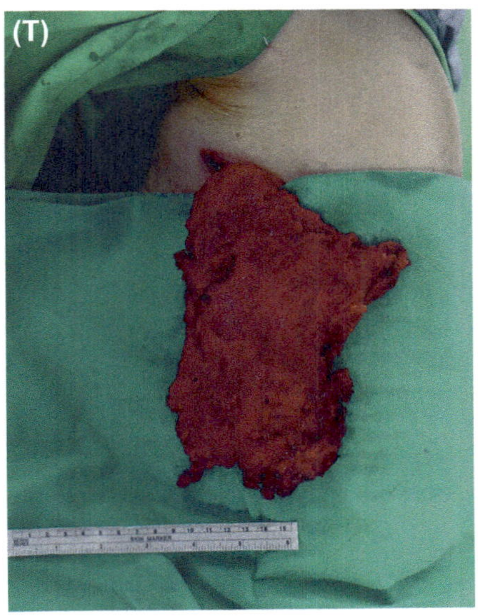

11.26T

Pedicled LD flap exteriorized.

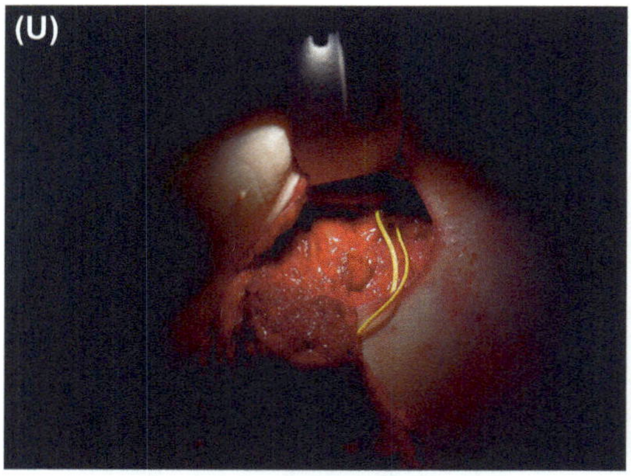

11.26U

Thoracodorsal bundle shown here (within vessel loop).

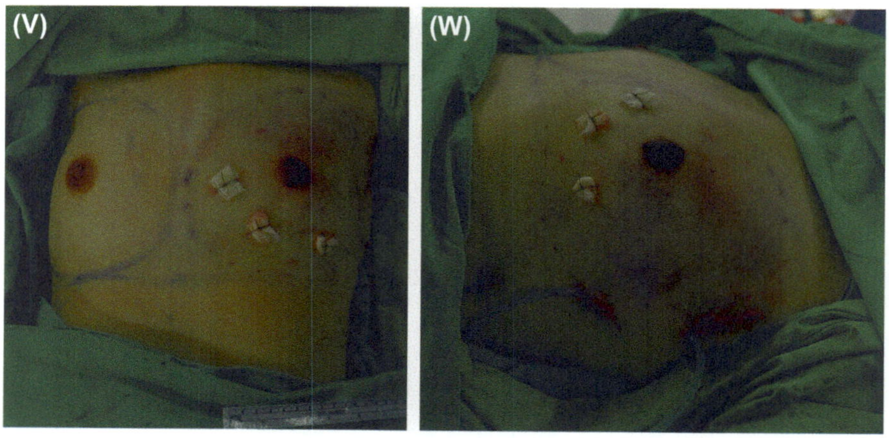

11.26V, W

Immediate on-table post-operative views.

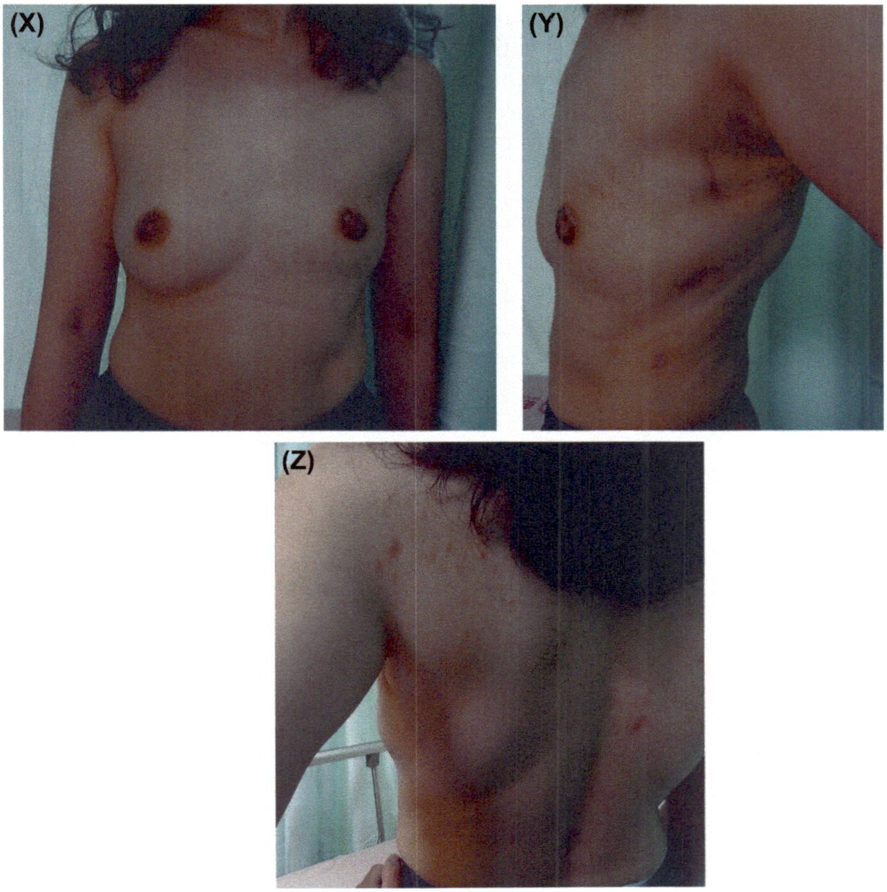

11.26X–Z

8 months post-operative view showing excellent cosmesis in terms of scar placement and satisfactory symmetry.

Discussion

The main advantage of performing pedicled LD flap harvest with robotic nipple-sparing mastectomy operation is that it can all be performed with only one small and inconspicuous axillary wound. This is a major plus point compared to conventional latissimus dorsi flap harvest which involves leaving a long donor site incision (Serra-Renom, Serra-Mestre, Martinez, D'Andrea, 2013). Other than cosmetically pleasing, avoidance of potential wound related morbidities is also an important consideration. In addition, with the extent of skin incision taken out of the picture, one could potentially harvest the maximal amount of flap without worrying about wound closure (Sood, Easow, Konopka, Panthaki, 2018). Disadvantages include the potentially long operative time and complexity of the procedures when performing both operations at the same sitting. In terms of patient selection, the authors believe that this reconstruction technique is most suitable for women with small to medium-sized breast with early breast cancer indicated for nipple-sparing mastectomy while desiring an autologous breast reconstruction (Lai et al., 2018).

References

Lai, H. W., & Lin, S. L. (2018). Robotic nipple sparing mastectomy and immediate breast reconstruction with robotic latissimus dorsi flap harvest – Technique and preliminary results. *Journal of Plastic, Reconstructive and Aesthetic Surgery.* https://doi.org/10.1016/j.bjps.2018.07.006.

Serra-Renom, J. M., Serra-Mestre, J. M., Martinez, L., & D'Andrea, F. (2013). Endoscopic reconstruction of partial mastectomy defects using latissimus dorsi muscle flap without causing scars on the back. *Aesthetic Plastic Surgery.* https://doi.org/10.1007/s00266-013-0192-3.

Sood, R., Easow, J. M., Konopka, G., & Panthaki, Z. J. (2018). Latissimus dorsi flap in breast reconstruction: Recent innovations in the workhorse flap. *Cancer Control.* https://doi.org/10.1177/1073274817744638.

CHAPTER

12

Endoscopic breast conserving surgery with immediate partial breast reconstruction using robot-assisted harvest of pedicled omental flap

Description of technique

Pre-operative marking and positioning

Pre-operative marking was done with the patient in standing and supine position. After induction of general anaesthesia, the patient was then placed in the supine position and ipsilateral arm abducted to 90 degrees to avoid affecting the operative procedure. Endoscopic video monitors (Olympus Optical Co., Tokyo, Japan) were set up on both sides of the patient's head to allow both the surgeon and the assistant to view the monitor. An oblique-ended rigid endoscope measuring 5 mm in diameter with a viewing angle of 30 degrees was used in all procedures.

Axillary staging procedure

In patients for whom sentinel lymph node biopsy (SLNB) is indicated, a small amount (2–3 mCi) of radioisotope Tc99m was injected intradermally at the site of the tumour before operation (either on the day or 1 day prior).

After induction of general anaesthesia, 3 mL of 1% methylene blue (Merck, Darmstadt, Germany) was injected into the breast parenchyma in equally divided aliquots at five positions surrounding the hemisphere of the tumour facing the ipsilateral axilla. The breast tissue from the tumour to the axilla was then gently massaged for 5–10 minutes. Within 20–30 minutes after injection of the blue dye, a handheld gamma probe (Navigator; USSC, Norwalk, CT) was used to identify the hot spots, and the location of the hottest nodes was then marked. An approximately 3-cm oblique axillary incision was then made close to the hottest nodes, and SLNB was then performed. Fresh frozen section was performed as indicated. If SLN was positive for metastases, a complete axillary lymph node dissection up to level II was performed.

Minimally Invasive (Endoscopic & Robotic) Breast Surgery. https://doi.org/10.1016/B978-0-323-73405-9.00012-1

Dissection of breast parenchyma off pectoralis major fascia

After completion of axillary staging procedure, dissection was carried out to the lateral border of the pectoralis major muscle. The margin between pectoralis muscle and breast parenchyma was clearly identified. An endoscopic Ultra Retractor (Johnson & Johnson KK or Karl Storz) vein harvester was used for the dissection pectoral muscle fascia off posterior portion of breast parenchyma. The penetrating vessels were coagulated and cut with bipolar scissors (PowerStar, Johnson & Johnson KK) or a harmonic scalpel to ensure adequate haemostasis and therefore better visual clarity. Counter traction was applied by retracting surrounding tissue with the Ultra Retractor under endoscopic guidance to create a sufficient working space, and a suction tube can be used to evacuate mist and smoke.

Tunnelling and development of skin flap

After completion of the axillary staging procedure, a semi-circular peri-areolar skin incision or an inframammary crease incision was made (depending on tumour location or surgeon's preference). A physiological saline solution containing lidocaine 0.05% and epinephrine 1:1,000,000 was injected subcutaneously into the whole breast to minimize bleeding. An approximately 3–5-mm-thick skin flap was created via tunnelling method using an optical bladeless trocar Xcel (Johnson & Johnson, Tokyo, Japan) under endoscopic guidance. Subsequently, the septa between the skin flap and parenchyma was dissected and taken off under endoscopic guidance using endoscissors, bipolar scissors, or a harmonic scalpel.

Performing wide excision

After development of adequate skin flap (either via a single axillary or combination of axillary and peri-areolar or inframammary incision), wide excision was performed using bipolar or monopolar diathermy. To guide resection with adequate margins, the authors recommended the use of intra-operative ultrasound and marking of resection margin with blue dye injection. Specimen was retrieved thereafter and haemostasis secured.

Robotic pedicled omental flap harvest and reconstruction

With patient placed in supine position, a 10-mm camera port was placed through an infraumbilical incision via open cutdown. Pneumoperitoneum was then created with CO_2 insufflation. Four working ports were then placed with two over the right lumbar region and two over the left. After gross inspection of the intra-abdominal cavity to ensure no abnormalities seen, omentum was identified and lifted up. Dissection of the omentum was performed slightly left to the centre of the transverse colon and advanced towards the splenic flexure using a Harmonic Ace Curved Shears (Ethicon Endo-Surgery Inc., Cincinnati, OH). Care must be taken to ligate and divide the left gastroepiploic vessels near the spleen. All other branches were divided as close to the stomach as possible. In a pedicled omental flap, the right gastroepiploic vessels were preserved as the feeding vessels for the flap and the dissection should stop right past the pyloric channel, after confirming preservation of the right gastroepiploic vessels. After isolation of the flap was completed, an approximately 2–3-finger breadths subcutaneous tunnel was prepared from the medial end of the inframammary fold (a new incision may be required if not through the same incision for wide excision) towards the xiphoid process till the linea alba was encountered. Thereafter, a 2–3 cm longitudinal incision was made on the linea alba and abdominal cavity entered to deliver the flap. Care must be taken to avoid twisting of pedicle. Securing the flap to the resection cavity with absorbable sutures was then performed at the end of the reconstruction. Drain was placed on a case-to-case basis or based on the surgeon's preference.

Case 27: endoscopic breast-conserving surgery with robot-assisted immediate pedicled omental flap reconstruction – hybrid technique

Patient/demographics

The case described a 37-year-old lady diagnosed with right breast cancer with a pre-operative core biopsy report of an invasive ductal carcinoma, ER+/PR+/CerbB2 negative performed at another institution. Pre-operative mammographic and sonographic evaluation showed two clusters of closely adhered microcalcifications as well as post-biopsy changes on sonographic imaging. Breast MRI showed an overall tumor size of 3.5cm in the right upper inner quadrant.

Her metastatic workup did not reveal any distant metastases.

After discussion regarding various treatment modalities, she opted for an endoscopic breast-conserving surgery with robot-assisted immediate pedicled omental flap reconstruction.

Surgery and pathology report

The patient underwent an endoscopic breast-conserving surgery, sentinel lymph node biopsy with robot-assisted immediate pedicled omental flap reconstruction. Sentinel lymph node biopsy was positive for metastases on the frozen section analysis; hence, the patient then proceeded to have an axillary dissection. Her final histology was reported as a T2N1M0, stage 2B, and she subsequently received adjuvant radiotherapy and endocrine therapy with Gonadotropin-releasing hormone agonist (GnRHa) and Tamoxifen.

Post-operative outcomes

Patient was noted to have partial necrosis of the omentum flap and this was managed with local wound care. She had subsequently completed her adjuvant radiotherapy and currently on endocrine therapy without disease recurrence.

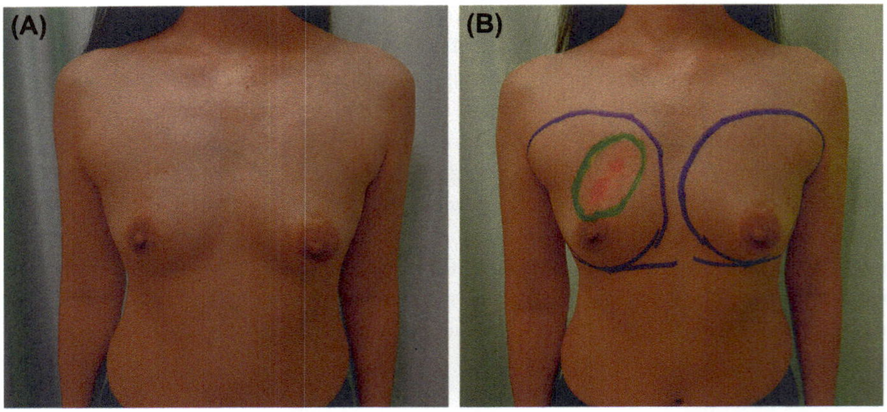

12.27A, B

Pre-operative views with markings showing tumor location and planned incisions.

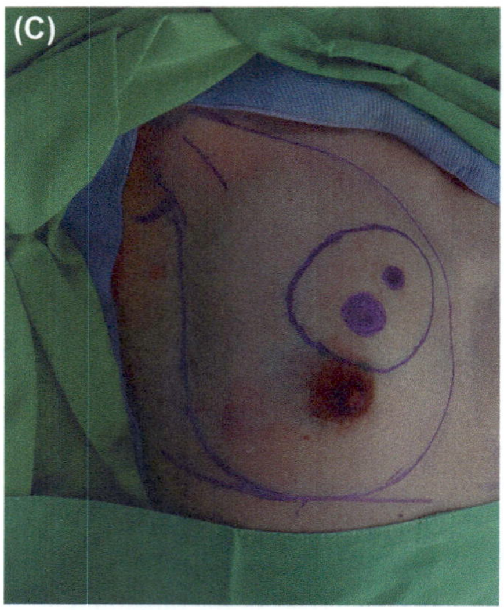

12.27C

On-table view showing planned incision.

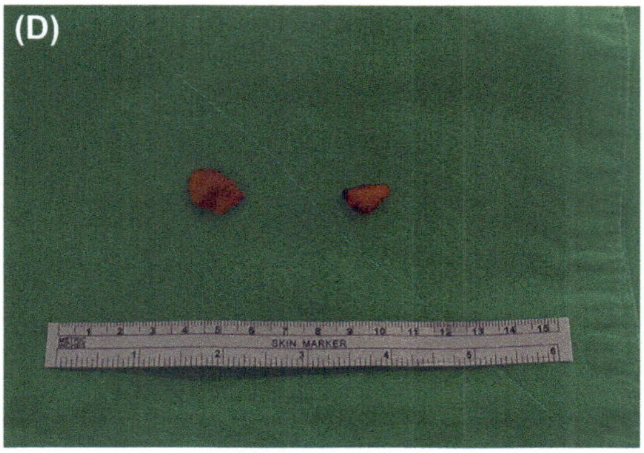

12.27D

Sentinel lymph nodes detected via dual modality.

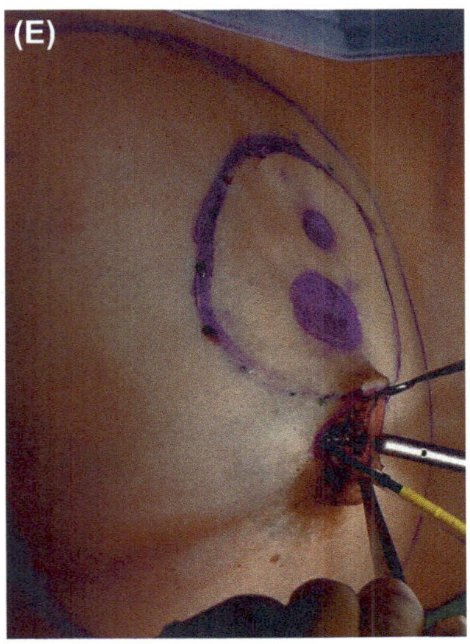

12.27E

Wide excision performed via peri-areolar incision.

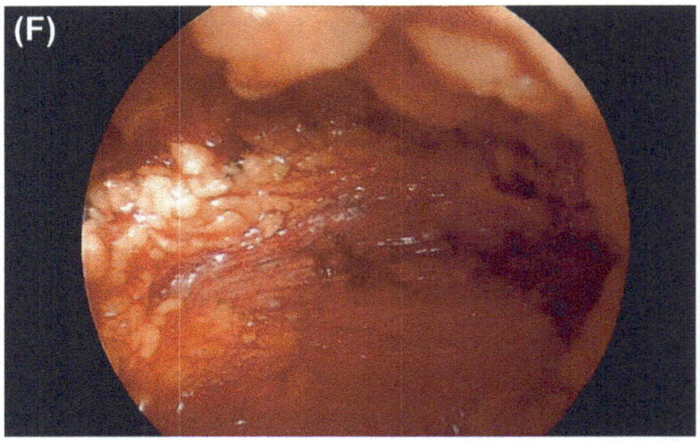

12.27F

Endoscopic view showing resection cavity after wide excision.

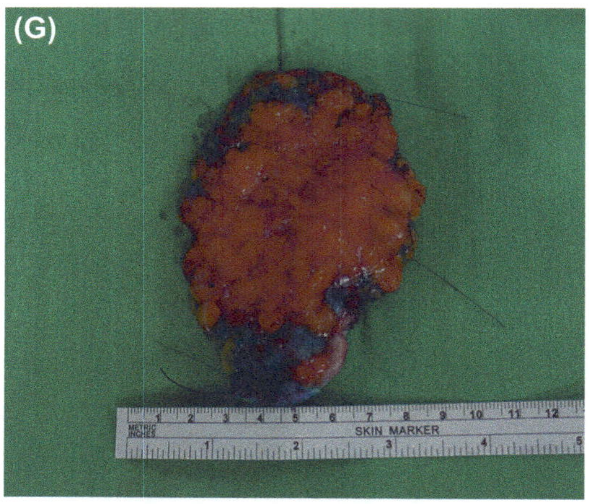

12.27G

Wide excision specimen removed intact and oriented.

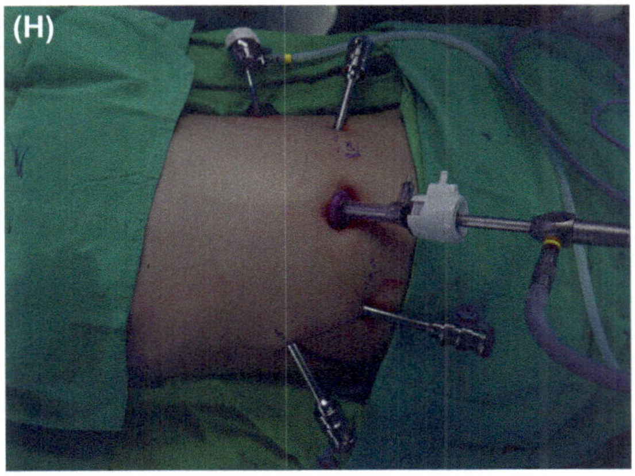

12.27H

Placement of camera and working ports as shown. Intra-abdominal cavity examined to ensure no gross abnormalities before proceeding with omental flap harvest.

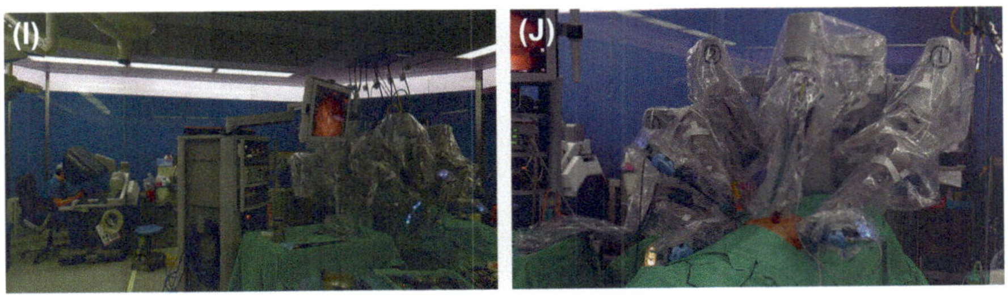

12.27I, J

Operating theater view showing the intra-operative setting, which was performed with a da Vinci Si (Intuitive Surgical, Sunnyvale, CA) robotic platform with the operating surgeon controlling at the surgeon's console. Robotic arms were placed as far as possible to avoid conflicts during operation.

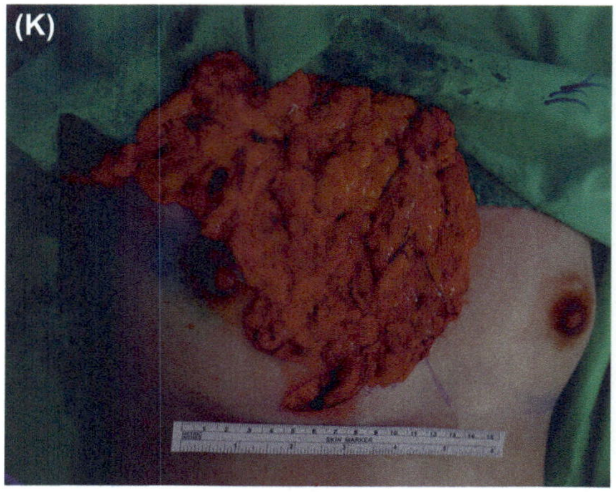

12.27K

Pedicled omental flap harvested and exteriorized.

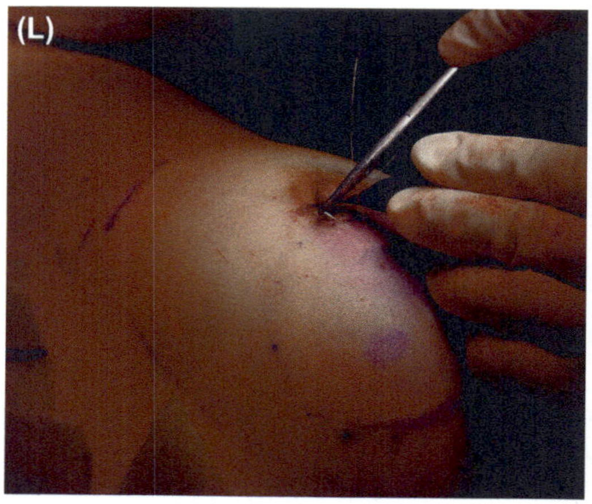

12.27L

Closure of inframammary crease and peri-areolar incisions.

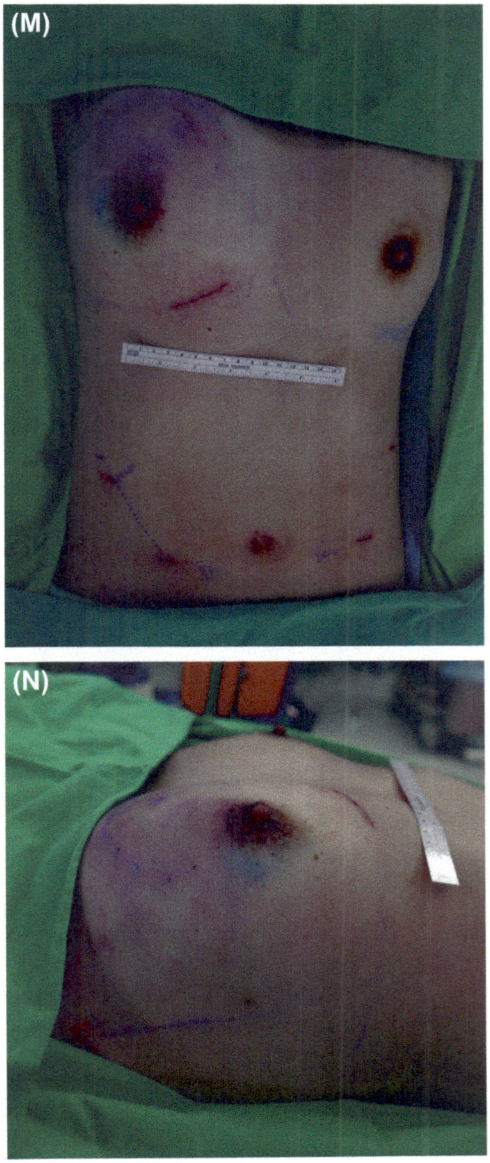

12.27M, N

Immediate post-operative views showing small incisions and good volume replacement.

Discussion

The main advantages of an omental flap include great versatility in terms of volume replacement, vascular reliability and most importantly, minimal donor-site morbidity. In terms of safety profile, omental flap has been proven to be generally safe as most cases in the literature healed without major complications (Zaha, Abe, Sagawa, Unesoko, 2017). Selection of patients suitable for this technique is not only limited to the lower quadrants during the initial phase of development (Zaha, 2015). Currently, the omental flap is versatile enough for volume replacement in any quadrants whether as free or pedicled flap. Medial-quadrant tissue defects, especially in the inner upper quadrant, which is known as 'no-man's land', are usually hard to repair and achieve good cosmesis but with omental flap, excellent cosmesis were reported. Although the omental flap harvest is not difficult, care has to be taken to ensure that patients are counselled regarding the possibility of inadequate volume for harvest and possible need for other options of reconstruction should there be inadequate omentum. There are no proven methods for pre-operative evaluation of omental volume and adequacy, and the authors suggested laparoscopy as the most definitive while remaining minimally invasive at the same time (Yi et al., 2017). Concerning the oncological safety of this technique (Westbroek & Douek, 2011), there were initial concerns of higher cancer or recurrence risks as several researchers have argued that adipocytes can stimulate the growth of breast cancer cells by increasing the local concentration of oestrogen, while some adipocytokines and the greater omentum may offer additional risks due to a high concentration of stem cells with great angiogenic potential. This theory, however, has not been proven by available clinical evidence.

References

Westbroek, D., & Douek, M. (2011). Laparoscopic harvest of omental flap for immediate breast reconstruction: An evolved modality for volume replacement. *European Journal of Surgical Oncology (EJSO)*. https://doi.org/10.1016/j.ejso.2011.08.030.

Yi, J., Zheng, Z., Li, J., Fan, J., Wang, T., Zhang, J., et al. (2017). Immediate breast reconstruction with omental flap for luminal breast cancer patients. *Medicine*. https://doi.org/10.1097/md.0000000000007797.

Zaha, H. (2015). Oncoplastic volume replacement technique for the upper inner quadrant using the omental flap. *Gland surgery*. https://doi.org/10.3978/j.issn.2227-684X.2015.01.08.

Zaha, H., Abe, N., Sagawa, N., & Unesoko, M. (2017). Oncoplastic surgery with omental flap reconstruction: A study of 200 cases. *Breast Cancer Research and Treatment*. https://doi.org/10.1007/s10549-017-4124-9.

CHAPTER

13 Minimally invasive breast surgery—A step-by-step graphic illustrations guide

Endoscopic breast conserving surgery—axilla incision

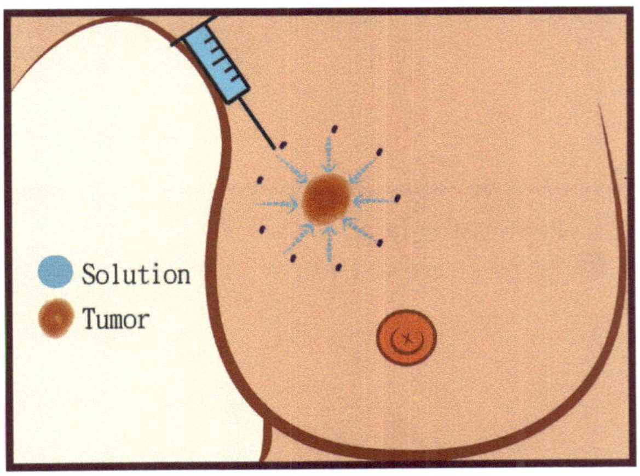

13.1

Injection of tumescence solution to aid in haemostasis and plane dissection.

Minimally Invasive (Endoscopic & Robotic) Breast Surgery. https://doi.org/10.1016/B978-0-323-73405-9.00013-3

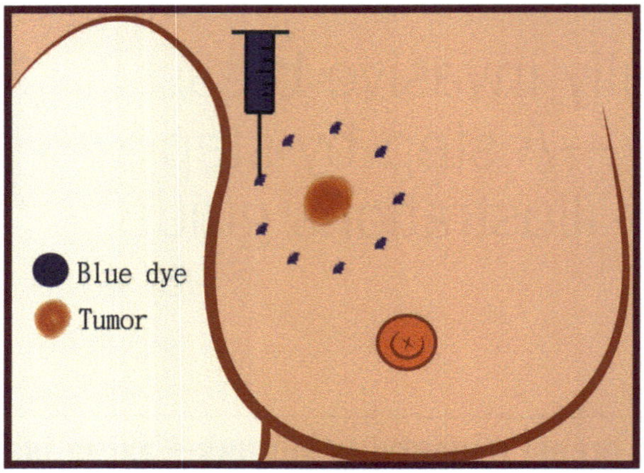

13.2

Injection of blue dye jelly (1 mL of methylene blue mixed with 10 mL of lignocaine or lidocaine jelly) to mark out margins of dissection.

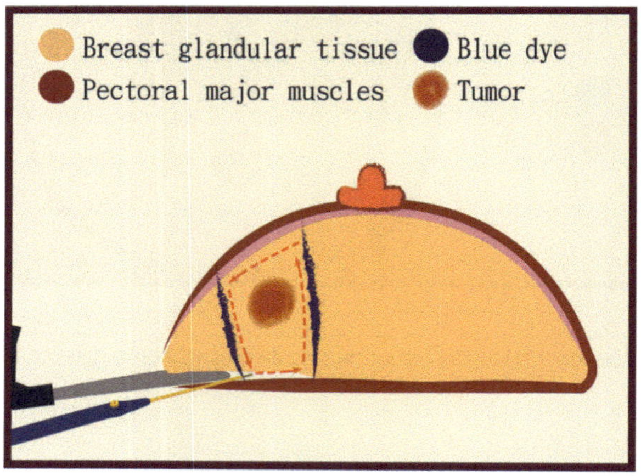

13.3

Dissection of posterior breast parenchyma off pectoralis major fascia with endoscopic vein harvester.

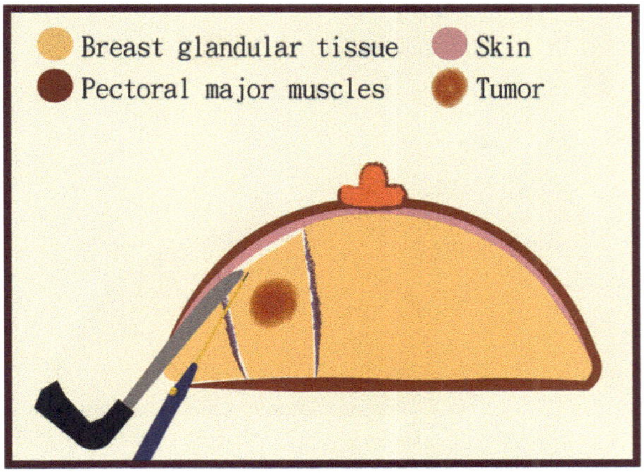

13.4

Dissection of anterior skin flap with endoscopic vein harvester.

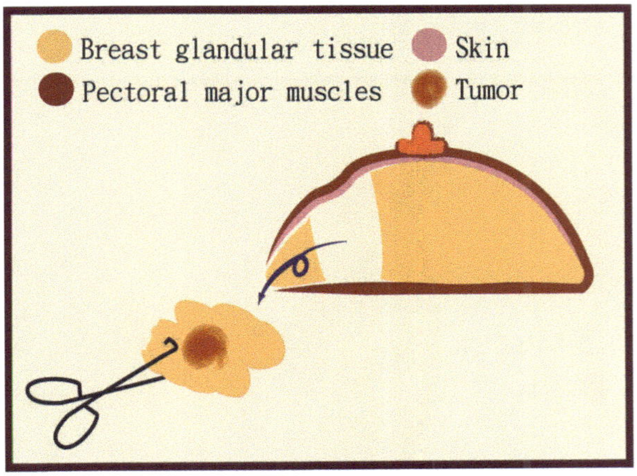

13.5

Retrieval of wide excision specimen.

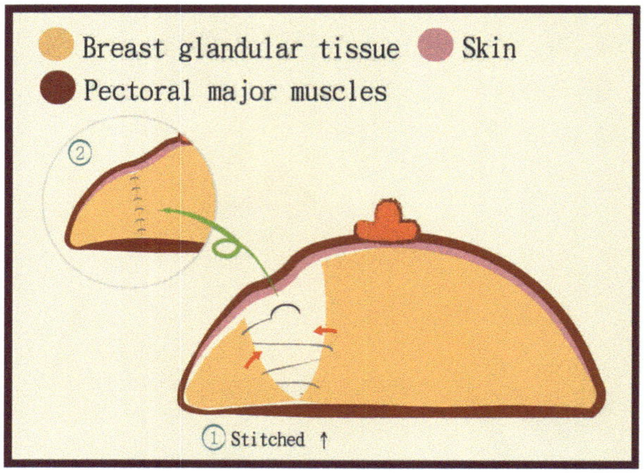

13.6

Approximation of breast parenchyma after wide excision.

Endoscopic breast conserving surgery—areolar incision

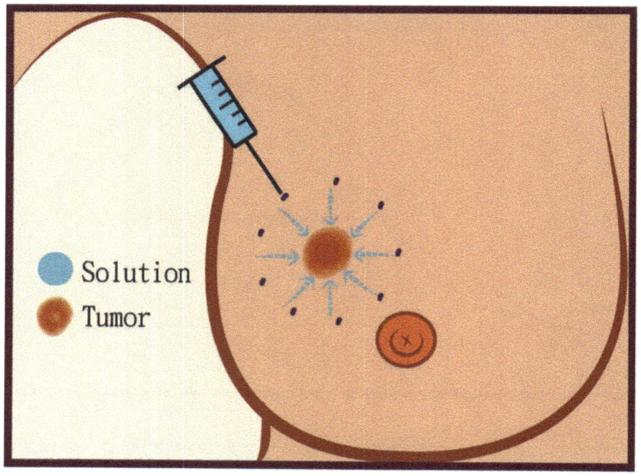

13.7

Injection of tumescence solution to aid in haemostasis and plane dissection.

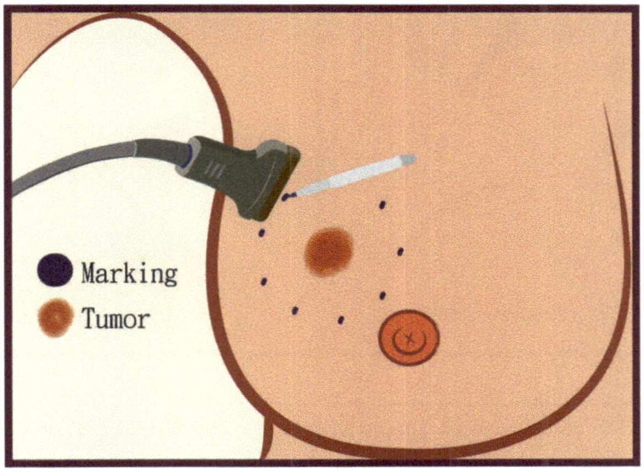

13.8

Intraoperative marking of margin with ultrasound.

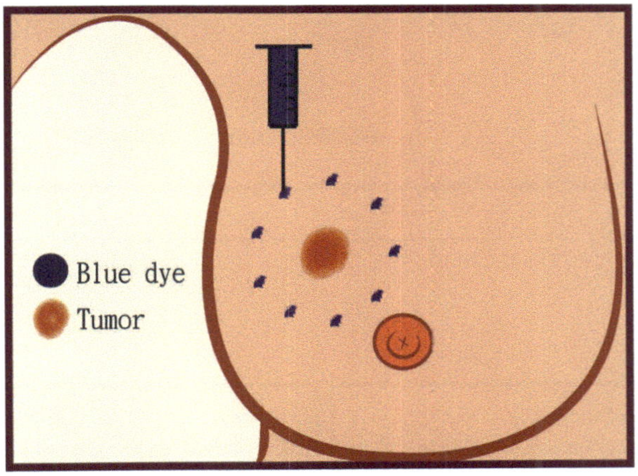

13.9

Injection of blue dye jelly (1 mL of methylene blue mixed with 10 mL of lignocaine or lidocaine jelly) to mark out margins of dissection.

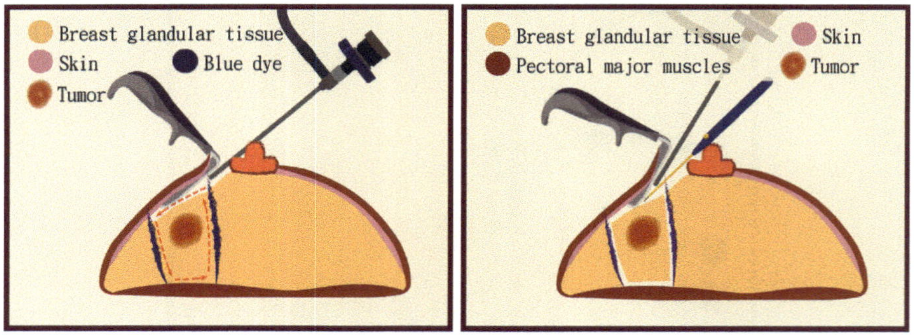

13.10, 13.11

Dissection of anterior skin flap with the aid of a 5 mm camera and lighted retractor.

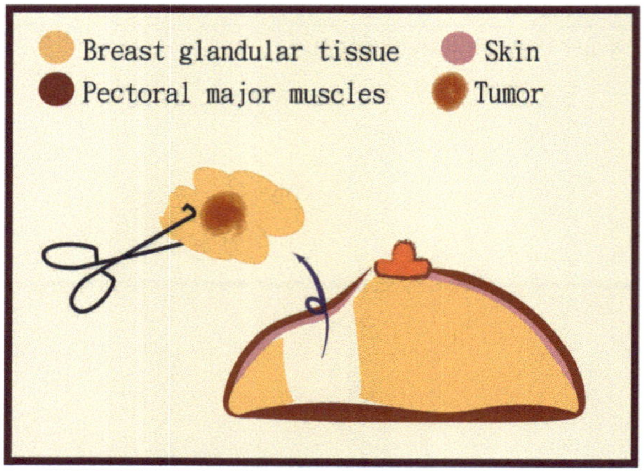

13.12

Retrieval of wide excision specimen.

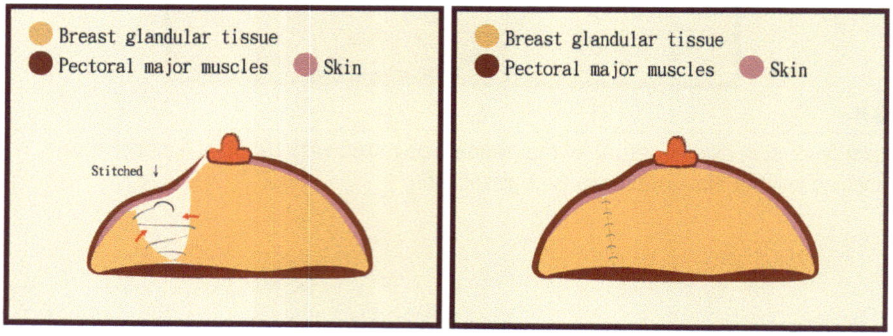

13.13, 13.14

Approximation of breast parenchyma after wide excision.

Endoscopic or robotic nipple sparing mastectomy with immediate implant reconstruction

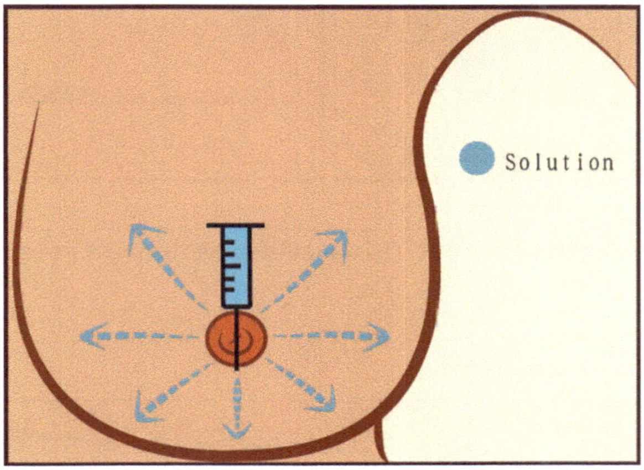

13.15

A physiological saline solution containing lidocaine 0.05% and epinephrine 1: 1,000,000 was injected subcutaneously into the whole breast to minimize bleeding.

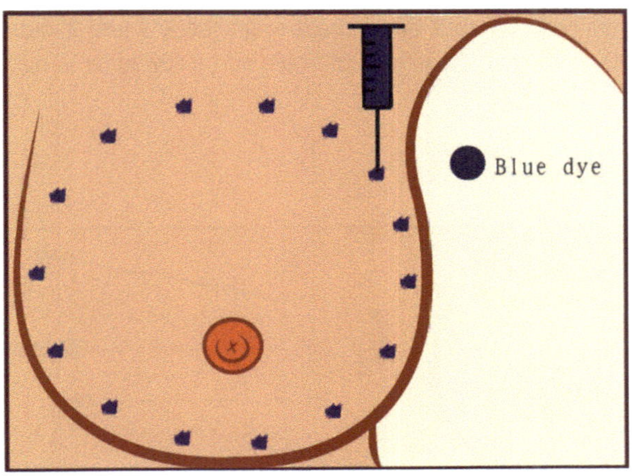

13.16

Injection of jelly containing methylene blue as a guide to mark the boundaries of resection.

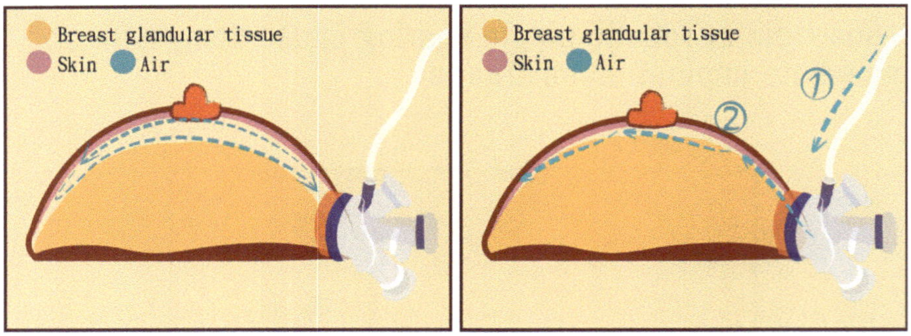

13.17, 13.18

After port placement, carbon dioxide (CO_2) was inflated with air pressure kept at 8 mmHg to create space for mastectomy.

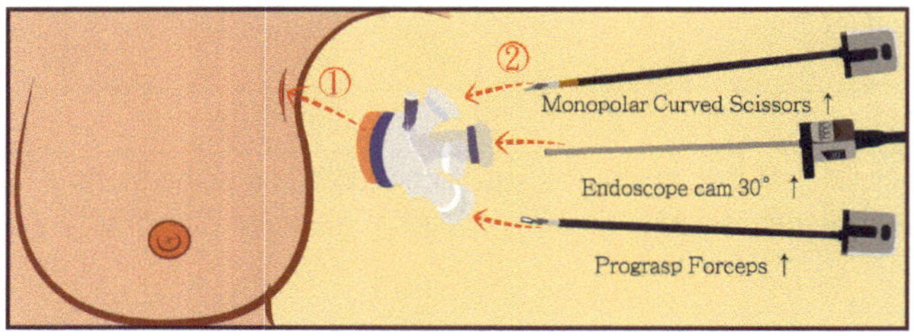

13.19

Illustration of insertion of single port and placement of instruments in robotic mastectomy (video camera, monopolar scissors, and forceps or grasper)."1 and 2' depicts the sequence or steps whereby: 1: placement of single port followed by 2: placement of instruments

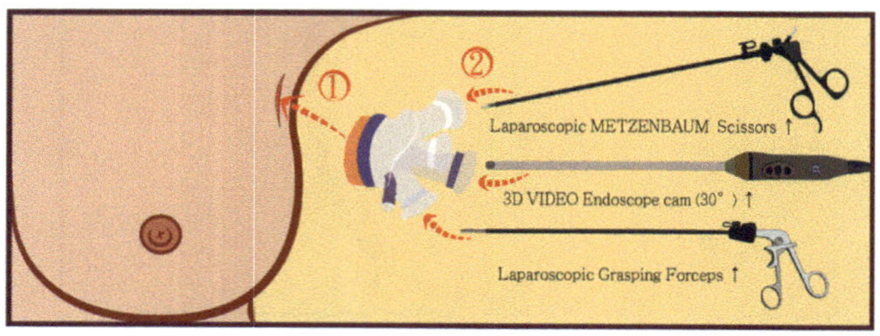

13.20

Illustration of insertion of single port and placement of instruments in single-port endoscopic mastectomy (video camera, laparoscopic Metzenbaum scissors, and laparoscopic grasping forceps).

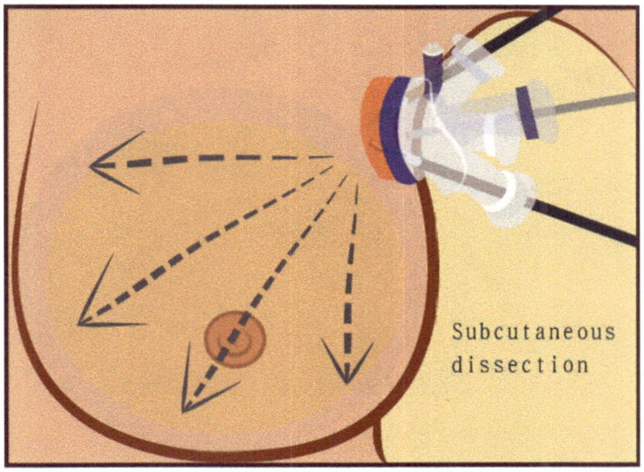

13.21

Dissection was commenced from the superficial skin flaps in all quadrants.

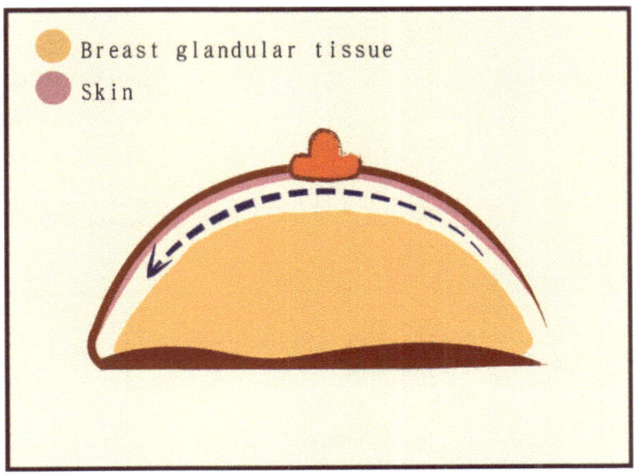

13.22

Dissection of subcutaneous skin flap.

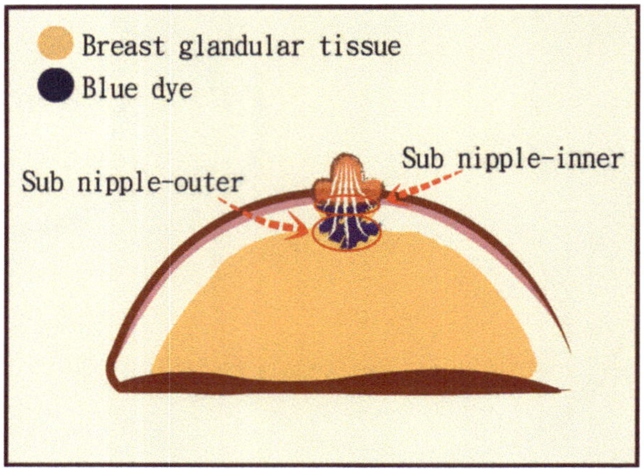

13.23

Intraoperative subnipple biopsies was performed and sent for frozen section analysis.

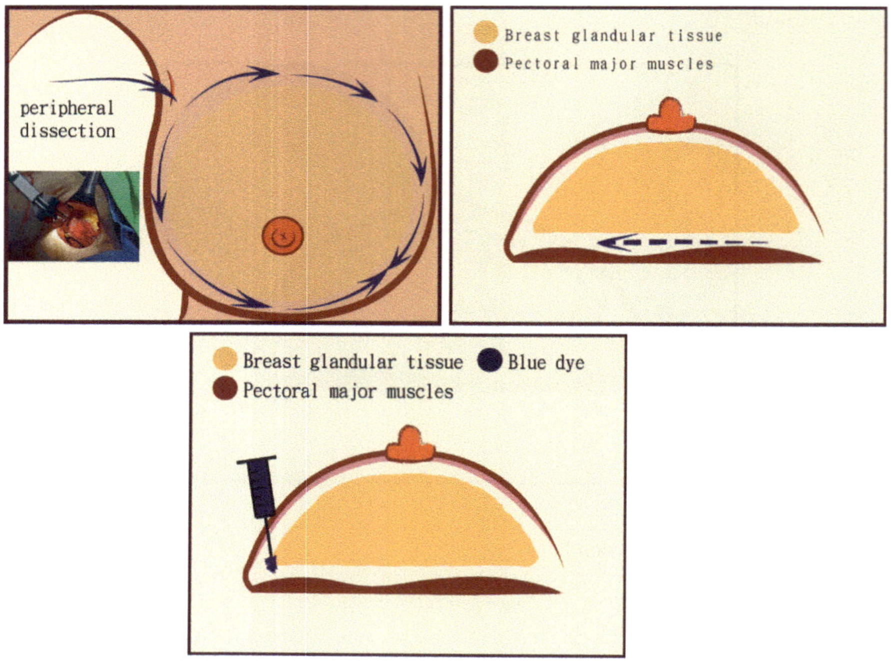

13.24–26

Peripheral and posterior dissection was performed with the guidance of the blue dye markings.

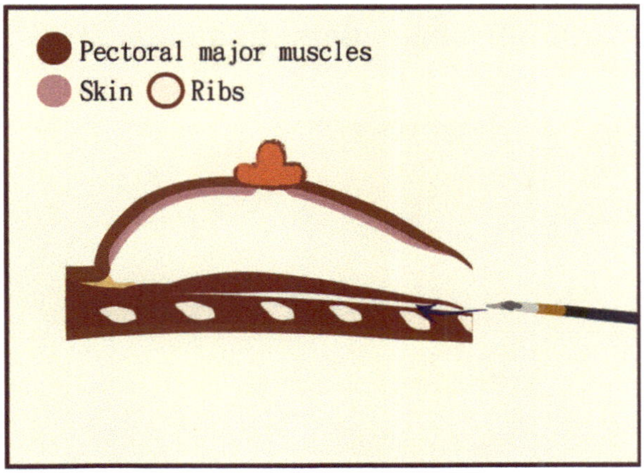

13.27

Breast reconstruction was performed with dissection of subpectoral muscular pocket.

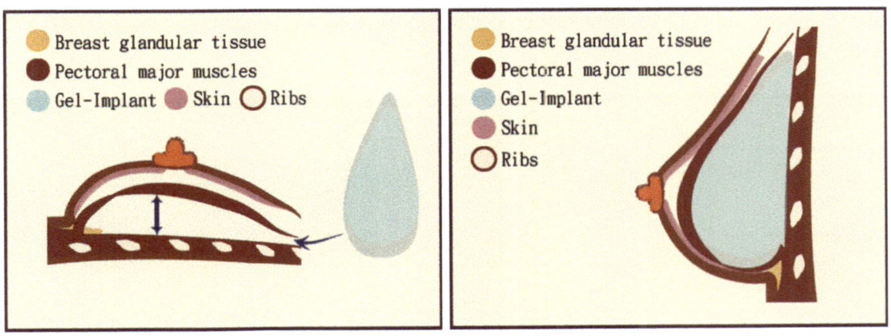

13.28, 13.29

Implant was placed via the axillary wound in the submuscular pocket.

Robotic assisted latissimus dorsi flap harvest

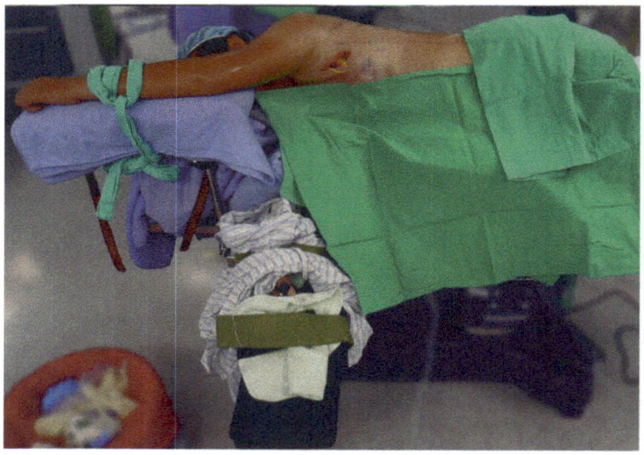

13.30

Patient positioning prior to commencement of robotic assisted latissimus dorsi (LD) flap harvest.

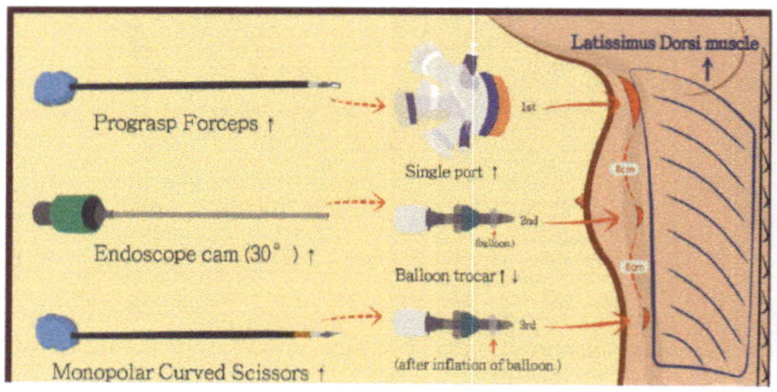

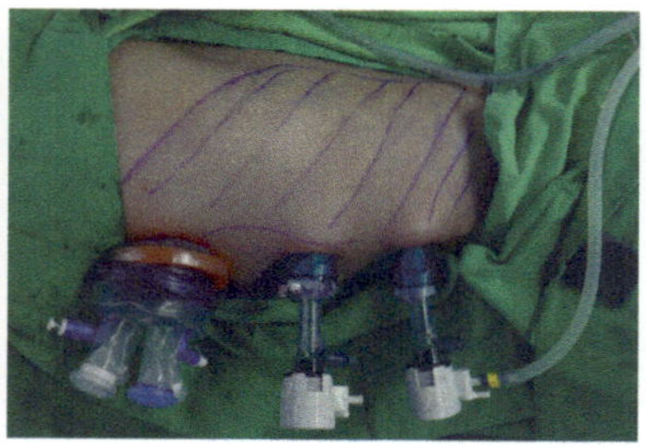

13.31, 13.32

Port and instruments positioning as shown (ProGrasp forceps through the single port over the axilla incision, video endoscope in the middle port, and monopolar scissors in the bottom port).

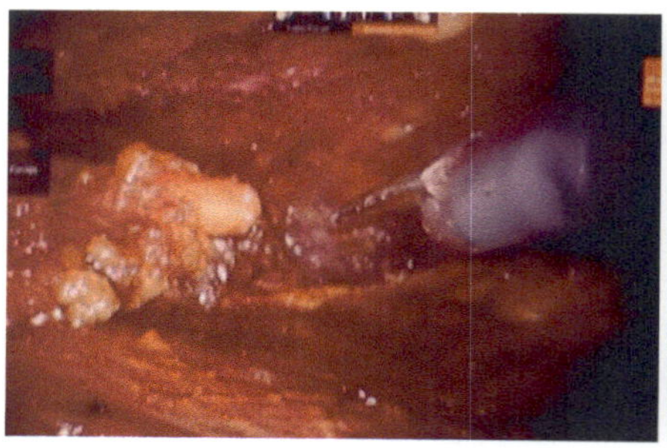

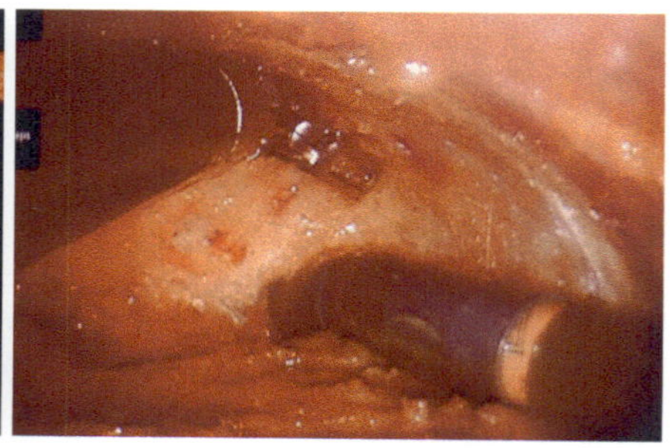

13.33, 13.34

Intraoperative view of flap harvest.

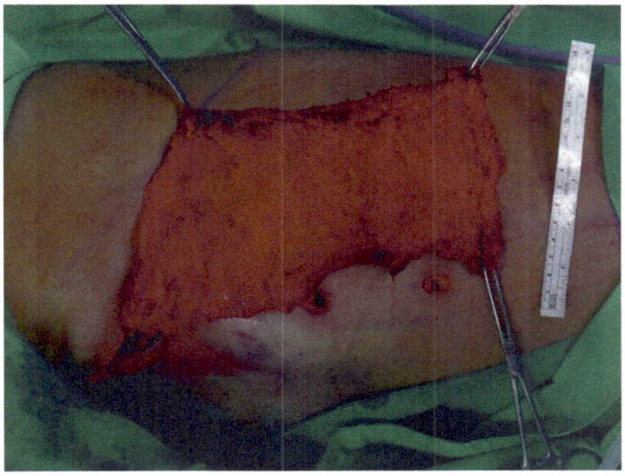

13.35

Pedicled latissimus dorsi (LD) flap completely exteriorized.

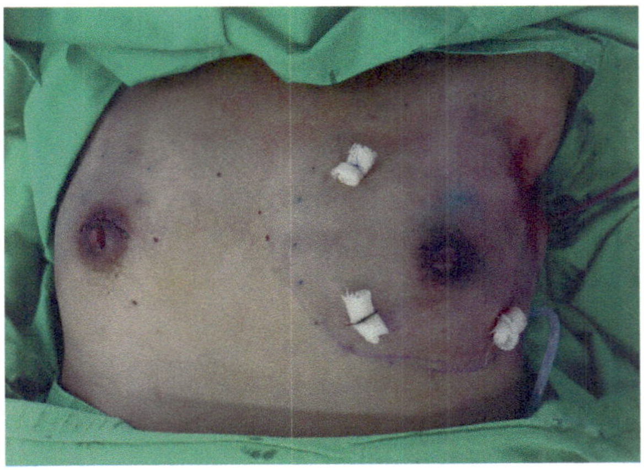

13.36

Immediate on-table postoperative view.

CHAPTER

Instruments used in minimally invasive breast surgery

14

Instruments in endoscopic breast conserving surgery

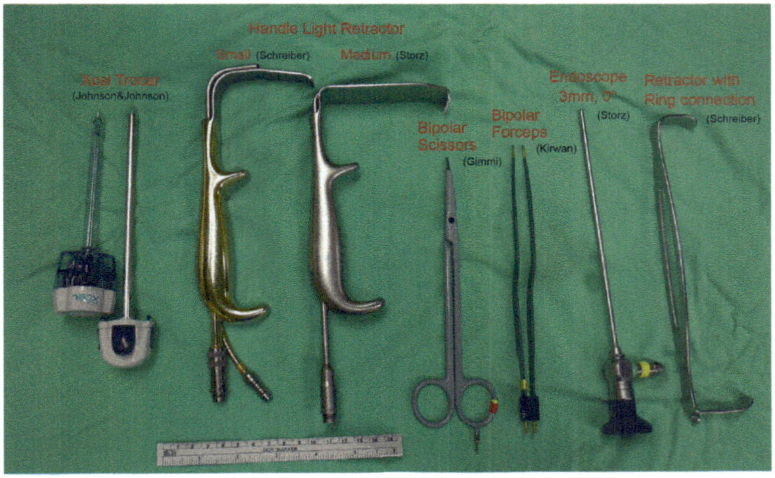

14.1

Common instruments used in endoscopic breast conserving surgery.

Minimally Invasive (Endoscopic & Robotic) Breast Surgery. https://doi.org/10.1016/B978-0-323-73405-9.00014-5

Instruments in endoscopic nipple-sparing mastectomy

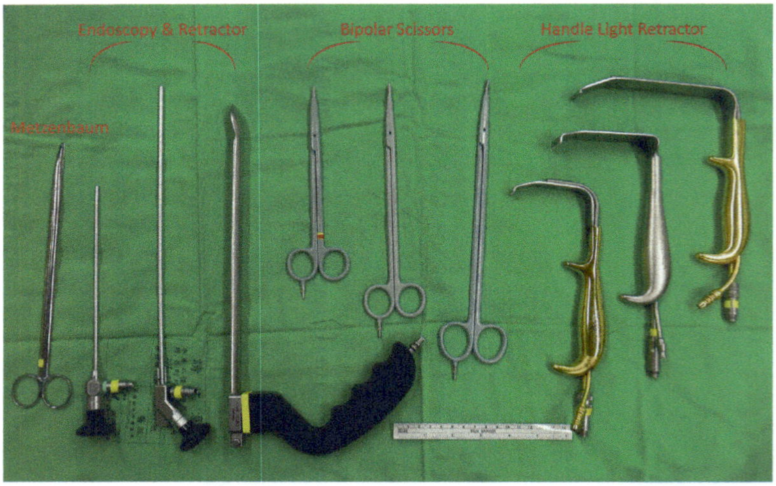

14.2

Common instruments used in endoscopic nipple sparing mastectomy.

Instruments in single port three-dimensional (3D) endoscopic nipple sparing mastectomy

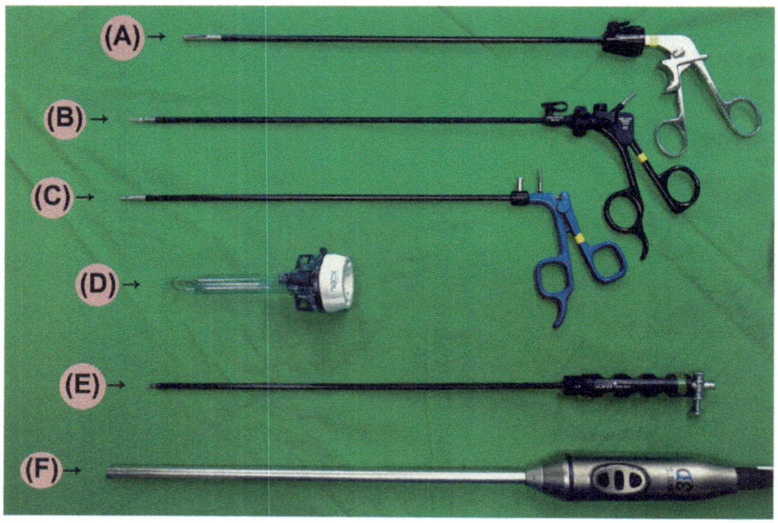

14.3

Common instruments used in endoscopic nipple-sparing mastectomy. (A) Laparoscopic grasping forceps. (B) Laparoscopic metzenbaum scissors. (C) Laparoscopic hook scissors. (D) 12 mm Endopath xcel bladeless trocar. (E) Laparoscopic suction coagulator with spatula tip. (F) 3D Video endoscope (30 degree).

Instruments in robotic nipple-sparing mastectomy (Si system)

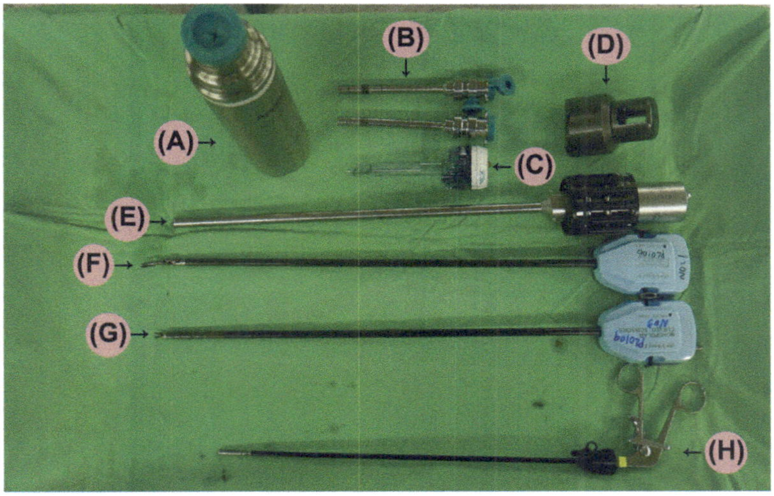

14.4

Common instruments used in robotic nipple sparing mastectomy (da Vinci Si System). (A) Scope warmer system. (B) 8 mm Instrument cannula. (C) 12 mm Endopath xcel Bladeless trocar. (D) Alignment target 12 mm endoscope. (E) 12 mm endoscope (30 degree). (F) 8 mm ProGrasp forceps. (G) 8 mm Monopolar curved scissors. (H) Dexon grasping forceps.

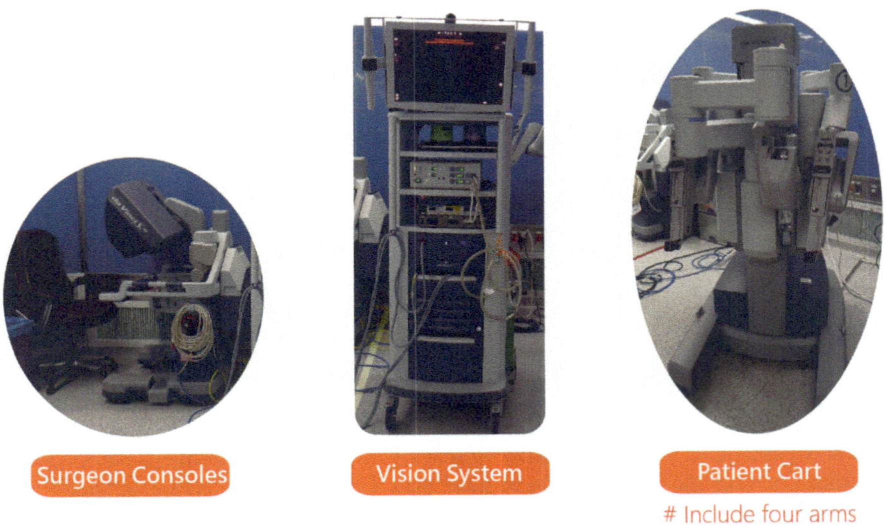

14.5

Da Vinci Si system (surgeon console, vision cart, and patient cart).

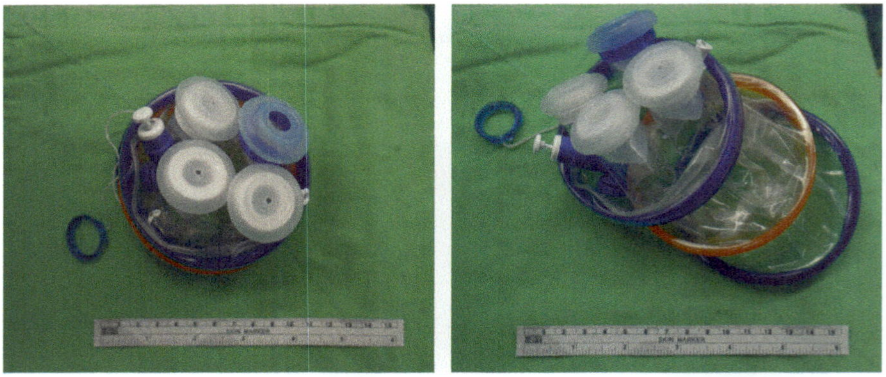

14.6

Single port system (Glove Port, Nelis, Gyeonggi-do, Korea).

Instruments in robotic nipple sparing mastectomy (Xi system)

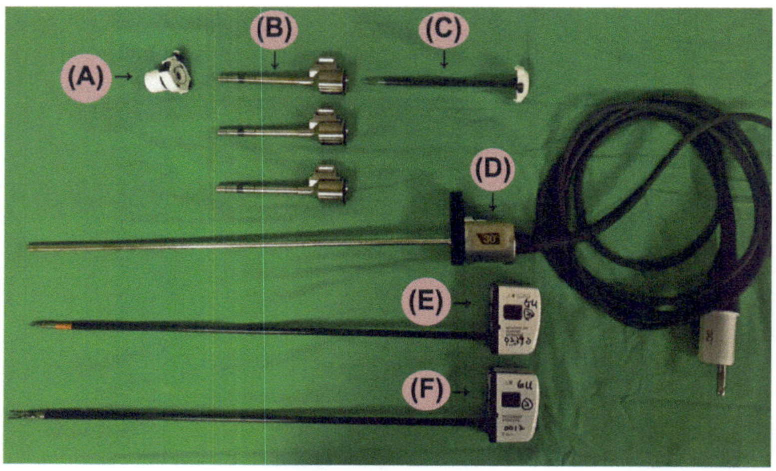

14.7

Common instruments used in robotic nipple sparing mastectomy (Da Vinci Xi system). (A) 5 -8 mm Universal seal. (B) 8 mm Instrument cannula. (C) 8 mm Bladeless obturator trocar. (D) 8 mm Endoscope with camera (30°). (E) 8 mm Monopolar curved scissors. (F) 8 mm Prograsp forceps.

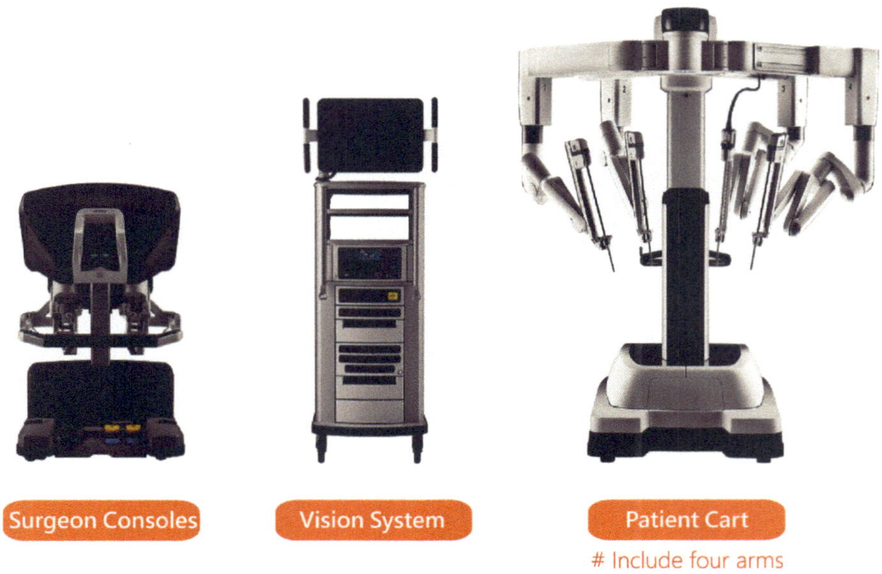

14.8

Da Vinci Xi system (surgeon console, vision cart, and patient cart).

Index

'*Note*: Page numbers followed by "f" indicate figures and "t" indicates tables.'

S

FSC
www.fsc.org
MIX
Papier | Fördert
gute Waldnutzung
FSC® C083411

Kolibri 360 GmbH
Ferdinand-Jühlke-Straße 7
99095 Erfurt, Deutschland
produktsicherheit@kolibri360.de